P9-CLZ-476

# STUDENT WORKBOOK
## TO ACCOMPANY
# Essentials of Human Diseases and Conditions

**third edition**

## Margaret Schell Frazier, RN, CMA, BS

*Retired*
Department Chair, Health and Human Services Division
Program Chair, Medical Assisting Program
Administrative Consultant Practitioner
Ivy Tech State College, Northeast
Fort Wayne, Indiana

Owner, Consultant
M & M Consulting
Hudson, Indiana

## Tracie Fuqua, CMA, BS

Program Director
Medical Assisting Program
Wallace State College
Hanceville, Alabama

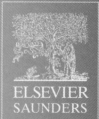

ELSEVIER
SAUNDERS

**ELSEVIER**
SAUNDERS

*An Imprint of Elsevier Science*

11830 Westline Industrial Drive
St. Louis, Missouri 63146

Student Workbook to Accompany
ESSENTIALS OF HUMAN DISEASES AND CONDITIONS          0-4160-0092-5

Third Edition

**Copyright © 2004 by Elsevier**

All rights reserved. No part of this publication may be reproduced or transmitted in any form
or by any means, electronic or mechanical, including photocopy, recording, or any information storage and retrieval system, without permission in writing from the publisher.

*Publishing Director:* Andrew Allen
*Executive Editor:* Adrianne Rippinger
*Senior Developmental Editor:* Rae L. Robertson
*Publishing Services Manager:* Linda McKinley
*Project Manager:* Julie Eddy
*Designer:* Julia Dummitt

Developing an understanding to disease processes is an exciting and fascinating facet of the health care provider's education. Considering that disease conditions are universally experienced, most of us have not only a natural curiosity about them, but as health care providers, it is essential that we are cognizant of the many components of disease. The study of current medical information on the more common clinical disorders encountered in the health care field presents a challenge to any student.

*Essentials of Human Diseases and Conditions,* third edition, attempts to condense and simplify current medical information on the more common clinical disorders encountered in the health field and physician office. This companion workbook is intended to present an orderly and concise review of information and to assist you in investigating diseases of the human body. The authors of this workbook, both medical-assisting educators and CMAs, recognize how essential it is for you to have an organized means of reinforcing and reviewing information presented in the text and during class sessions. It is our goal to provide a tool that will bolster the educational experience as you study pathophysiology, as well as to help you approach learning the basics of the human pathologic condition.

Students have previously expressed their desire to have a workbook or study guide to help with studying notes and preparing for examinations. This workbook is a means to review pertinent information, making it more likely that you will remember diseases along with their signs, symptoms, and treatments.

This workbook has been planned to follow the textbook chapters in an orderly fashion. Each chapter of the workbook follows the body systems and presents the review material in the following order:
- Word Definitions
- Glossary Terms
- Short Answer
- Fill-in-the-Blank
- Anatomical Structures
- Patient Screening
- Patient Teaching
- Essay Question
- Certification Exam Review (Multiple Choice)

## WORD DEFINITIONS

The sections titled *Word Definitions* list essential words to help you develop and understand disease entities. The use of a medical dictionary or medical terminology book may be necessary to arrive at the correct meaning of each word as it is used in the textbook.

## GLOSSARY TERMS

Glossary terms are boldfaced and/or italicized in each chapter and presented in the glossary section in the back of the textbook. It is suggested that you attempt to recall the information presented in class lecture and then confirm the definition with the textbook glossary.

## SHORT ANSWER

Short-answer questions are included in each chapter as a method of providing you with a means of recall. These questions address pertinent facts of selected diseases discussed in the chapter.

## FILL-IN-THE-BLANK

Fill-in-the-blank questions provide an opportunity for you to apply one-word or short answers, again to help reinforce and review the information presented. Answers are provided in *Word Lists* for rapid recognition.

## ANATOMICAL STRUCTURES

Illustrations of anatomical structures and processes are included for labeling. Knowledge of anatomy is crucial to understanding the concepts of disease processes. These labeling exercises are intended to enhance learning.

## PATIENT SCREENING

Selected patient-screening scenarios are presented to enable you to relate how you would handle telephone calls to the medical office. For these exercises, you should apply the following general guidelines for patient screening in combination with critical thinking skills to formulate a typical screening response. Five typical phone calls are presented per chapter.

## GUIDELINES FOR PATIENT-SCREENING EXERCISES

Typically, the medical assistant has the responsibility of screening telephone calls from patients requesting an appointment or reporting treatment progress or lack of progress. The medical assistant is often the initial contact for the patient or patient's family, and critical thinking and a prompt response are required. Many offices have established guidelines regarding the extent of assessment that can be made over the telephone in compliance with state practice acts. It is *essential* that office staff be aware of and follow office guidelines. Additionally, the medical assistant who is answering the phone may have a list of questions that he or she is expected to ask along with suggestions for appropriate responses regarding appointments or acceptable referrals. Important guidelines for life-threatening situations are listed in the textbook and in this workbook.

It is recommended that you review the information in the text regarding patient screening. The guidelines listed are not intended for diagnosing a caller's medical condition or for providing curative advice. These exercises offer *general clues* to enable you to recognize the urgency for an appointment, to identify individuals reporting an emergency, and to discern the kind of calls that require referral to the physician for response. These exercises are not intended to focus on the skill of medical triage, which state practice acts generally reserve for certain licensed professionals. When a patient calls, careful listening is essential because the caller often relays information that will help the medical assistant to decide the appropriate action required. Ideally, the outcome of telephone communication between caller and screener will benefit the patient and avoid potential medical and legal problems. The importance of sensitivity to human suffering, strict confidentiality, and a keen awareness of the priority of meeting the needs of patients are necessary skills of the telephone screener and cannot be overstated. The medical assistant must always keep in mind the following important facts:

- Only *physicians* and *nurse practitioners* may diagnose disease and prescribe medications.
- Established office protocol must *always* be followed during the screening process.
- All calls and referrals must be documented according to office policy.

The following list of serious and life-threatening conditions require immediate assessment and intervention:

- Sudden onset of unexplained shortness of breath
- Crushing pain across the center of the chest
- Difficult breathing occurring suddenly and rapidly worsening, often in the middle of the night
- Vomiting bright red or very dark "coffee-grounds"–appearing blood

- Sudden onset of weakness and unsteadiness or severe dizziness
- Sudden loss of consciousness or paralysis
- Flashes of light in field of vision
- Sudden and progressively worsening abdominal, flank, or pelvic pain
- Sudden onset of blurred vision accompanied by severe throbbing in the eye
- Children and other individuals with a history of asthma and sudden onset of difficulty breathing

Additional symptoms requiring prompt assessment include but are not limited to:

- Sudden or recent onset of unexplained bleeding including blood in urine, stool, or emesis
- Coughing or spitting up of blood
- Unusual and unexplained or heavy vaginal bleeding
- Elevated body temperature of sudden onset or for a prolonged period
- Continued abdominal, back, or pelvic pain
- Sudden onset of headache-type pain
- Children with elevated temperatures or continued vomiting
- Infants with sudden onset of projectile vomiting

It is essential to document all calls according to office policy and to notify the physician in an emergency situation.

# PATIENT TEACHING

Selected patient-teaching scenarios are included to enable you to convey how you would handle patient-teaching opportunities in the medical office. For these exercises, you should apply the following general guidelines for patient teaching.

## GUIDELINES FOR PATIENT-TEACHING EXERCISES

These exercises are intended to provide you with an opportunity to develop patient-teaching skills. The actual implementation of these skills is dependent on state practice acts and office policies. You have the responsibility to make yourself aware of your state's practice acts and office policy before attempting actual patient teaching. Once you have ascertained that patient teaching is within your scope of practice, you should check office policy for suggested protocol. Many offices have established guidelines for patient teaching, as well as printed materials to assist the health care professional in patient-teaching responsibilities.

- Most offices have patient instructions that are written on the encounter form at the end of the physician's contact with the patient.
- As the patient signs out or before he or she leaves the examination room, the medical assistant reviews these instructions with the patient.
- Often the scheduling of a return visit is the only instruction the physician may write.

Other identified instructions may be the scheduling of additional testing or the inclusion of information about diets or prescribed medications. Although these instructions are a form of patient teaching, reinforcing patient instructions and obtaining patient feedback that confirms his or her understanding of the instructional material is usually considered an essential responsibility for any health care provider. You are encouraged to review general principles of patient teaching as provided in the text.

- It is important to remember that the patient is a partner in health care and that patient teaching, as an ongoing process, requires interaction with the patient and his or her family or caregiver.
- Presenting the material to the patient must be done at the patient's level of understanding.

As you approach each patient-teaching experience, you should have a goal in mind. Usually patients will express goals for a recovery or improvement in their health situation during the intake assessment procedure. Encouraging input from the patient and family or caregiver in setting goals and delegating responsibility for suggested procedures or activities are in the best interest of the patient. The development of a trusting relationship and effective communication helps because individuals are encouraged to assume responsibility for their health and recovery.

The patient-teaching scenarios provided are possible patient-teaching opportunities for the health care professional. The scenarios are presented for every chapter except Chapter 1. You should describe how you would approach the appropriate teaching activity for each situation. Certain patient-teaching opportunities could be duplicated because many teaching concepts are generalized for similar conditions. Once wound care has been explained, it is not necessary for you to repeat this type of instruction in a detailed manner in similar scenarios. Daily weights and requirements for taking medications at the same time every day are examples of patient-teaching opportunities that apply to many patient-teaching situations. Handwashing reminders are an important factor to be mentioned in most teaching opportunities.

# Essay Questions

One essay question is included for each chapter. These questions will provide you with an opportunity to discuss or explain in detail certain disease-related topics presented in the chapter.

# Certification Examination Review

Multiple choice–style questions simulate the typical format found in the certification examination. These questions are incorporated to prepare students for what they will encounter in the certification examination.

It is our goal to furnish you with the optimal study instruments to achieve an understanding of the disease entities you may encounter in a physician's office. We wish you success in your endeavor.

*Margaret Schell Frazier, RN, CMA, BS*
*Tracie Fuqua, CMA, BS*

**CHAPTER 2**

Unn Fig 2-1 (Circulation patterns before and after birth) *From Applegate EJ:* The anatomy and physiology learning system, *2 ed, Philadelphia, 2000, Saunders.*

Unn Fig 2-2, *A* (Ventricular septal defect) *Used with permission of Ross products Division, Abbott Laboratories; from* Congenital Heart Abnormalities *(Clinical Education Aid no 7, 1992.*

**CHAPTER 5**

Unn Fig 5-2 (The visual pathway) *From Gould B:* Pathophysiology for the health professions, *2 ed, Philadelphia, 2000, Saunders.*

**CHAPTER 6**

Unn Fig 6-1 (Normal skin) *From Patton KT, Thibodeau GA:* Mosby's handbook of anatomy & physiology, *St Louis, 2000, Mosby.*

**CHAPTER 8**

Unn Fig 8-1 (Main and accessory organs of the normal digestive system) *Redrawn from Miller M:* Pathophysiology: principles of disease, *Philadelphia, 1983, Saunders.*

**CHAPTER 10**

Unn Fig 10-1 (Anterior view of the heart) *From Patton KT, Thibodeau GA:* Mosby's handbook of anatomy & physiology, *St Louis, 2000, Mosby.*

Unn Fig 10-2 (Posterior view of the heart) *From Patton KT, Thibodeau GA:* Mosby's handbook of anatomy & physiology, *St Louis, 2000, Mosby.*

Unn Fig 10-3 (Cardiac cycle) *From Gould B:* Pathophysiology for the health professions, *2 ed, Philadelphia, 2000, Saunders.*

Unn Fig 10-3 (Layers of the heart wall) *From Applegate EJ:* The anatomy and physiology learning system, *2 ed, Philadelphia, 2000, Saunders.*

**CHAPTER 11**

Unn Fig 11-1 (Gross anatomy of the urinary) *From Gould B:* Pathophysiology for the health professions, *2 ed, Philadelphia, 2000, Saunders.*

Unn Fig 11-2 (Internal structure of the kidney) *From Gould B:* Pathophysiology for the health professions, *2 ed, Philadelphia, 2000, Saunders.*

Unn Fig 11-3 (The nephron) *From Patton KT, Thibodeau GA:* Mosby's handbook of anatomy & physiology, *St Louis, 2000, Mosby.*

Unn Fig 11-4 (Formation of urine) *From Gould B:* Pathophysiology for the health professions, *2 ed, Philadelphia, 2000, Saunders.*

**CHAPTER 13**

Unn Fig 13-1 (Normal brain) *From Gould B:* Pathophysiology for the health professions, *2 ed, Philadelphia, 2000, Saunders.*

Unn Fig 13-2 (Spinal cord) *From Gould B:* Pathophysiology for the health professions, *2 ed, Philadelphia, 2000, Saunders.*

Unn Fig 13-3 (Neuron) *From Gould B:* Pathophysiology for the health professions, *2 ed, Philadelphia, 2000, Saunders.*

Unn Fig 13-4 (Functional areas of the brain) *From Gould B:* Pathophysiology for the health professions, *2 ed, Philadelphia, 2000, Saunders.*

Unn Fig 13-7 (Autonomic nervous) *From Bonewit-West K:* Clinical procedures for medical assistants, *6 ed, Philadelphia, 2004, Saunders.*

Copyright ©2004, Elsevier. All rights reserved.

# Contents

# Mechanisms of Disease, Diagnosis, and Treatment

## WORD DEFINITIONS

*Define the following basic medical terms:*

1. Adipose — *fatty tissue*
2. Alopecia — *hair loss*
3. Analgesic —
4. Cognitive —
5. Dysfunction —
6. Ectopic — *abnormal position*
7. Endometrial —
8. Genetic — *relating to genes*
9. Hematopoietic — *actively dividing cells*
10. Hypervitaminosis — *too much vitamins*
11. Nosocomial — *pertaining to hospital*
12. Palliative —
13. Preoperatively —
14. Reflexology — *study of reflexes*
15. Systemic — *whole body*
16. Transcutaneous — *pertaining to the skin*
17. Transient — *lasting for a short term*
18. Urticaria — *hives*
19. Visceral — *internal*

Copyright ©2004, Elsevier. All rights reserved.

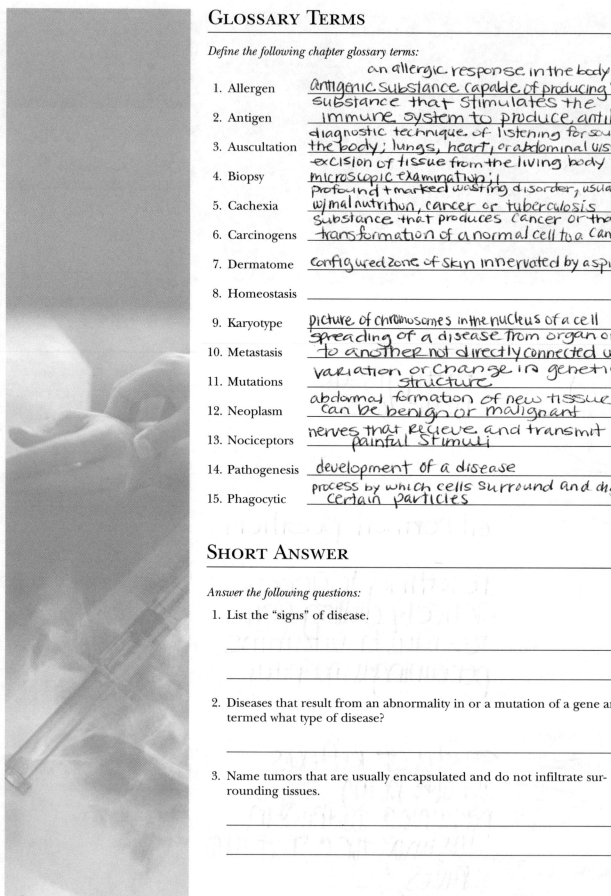

# GLOSSARY TERMS

*Define the following chapter glossary terms:*

1. Allergen — Antigenic substance capable of producing *an allergic response in the body*

2. Antigen — substance that stimulates the immune system to produce antibodies

3. Auscultation — diagnostic technique of listening for sounds w/in the body; lungs, heart, or abdominal viscera

4. Biopsy — excision of tissue from the living body followed by microscopic examination; I

5. Cachexia — profound + marked wasting disorder, usually associated w/ malnutrition, cancer or tuberculosis

6. Carcinogens — substance that produces cancer or that causes transformation of a normal cell to a cancerous one

7. Dermatome — configured zone of skin innervated by a spinal cord segment

8. Homeostasis — 

9. Karyotype — picture of chromosomes in the nucleus of a cell

10. Metastasis — spreading of a disease from organ or part to another not directly connected with it.

11. Mutations — variation or change in genetic structure

12. Neoplasm — abnormal formation of new tissue; can be benign or malignant

13. Nociceptors — nerves that recieve and transmit painful stimuli

14. Pathogenesis — development of a disease

15. Phagocytic — process by which cells surround and digest certain particles

# SHORT ANSWER

*Answer the following questions:*

1. List the "signs" of disease.

2. Diseases that result from an abnormality in or a mutation of a gene are termed what type of disease?

3. Name tumors that are usually encapsulated and do not infiltrate surrounding tissues.

Copyright ©2004, Elsevier. All rights reserved.

4. Name tumors with invasive cells that multiply excessively and infiltrate other tissues that can represent a serious threat to the patient.

_____

_____

5. Identify the hormone that may be elevated when a patient has prostate cancer.

_____

6. Cite the statistics for cancer deaths in the United States as estimated by the American Cancer Association.

_____

7. Any substance that causes an allergic response in a patient is called what?

_____

8. Identify the type of care that is focused on family support and comfort during terminal illness.

_____

9. At what age are patients encouraged to have annual physical examinations and screening tests to detect possible health problems?

_____

10. What may be the cause of immunodeficiency disorders?

_____

11. Name the part of the brain that is responsible for interpreting pain.

_____

12. What information is valuable in helping a health care provider assess a patient's condition?

_____

_____

13. What may the physician order to assist with the diagnosis of a patient?

_____

14. List examples of systemic manifestations of severe allergic responses.

_____

_____

15. List some examples of predisposing factors related to lifestyle.

_____

_____

Copyright ©2004, Elsevier. All rights reserved.

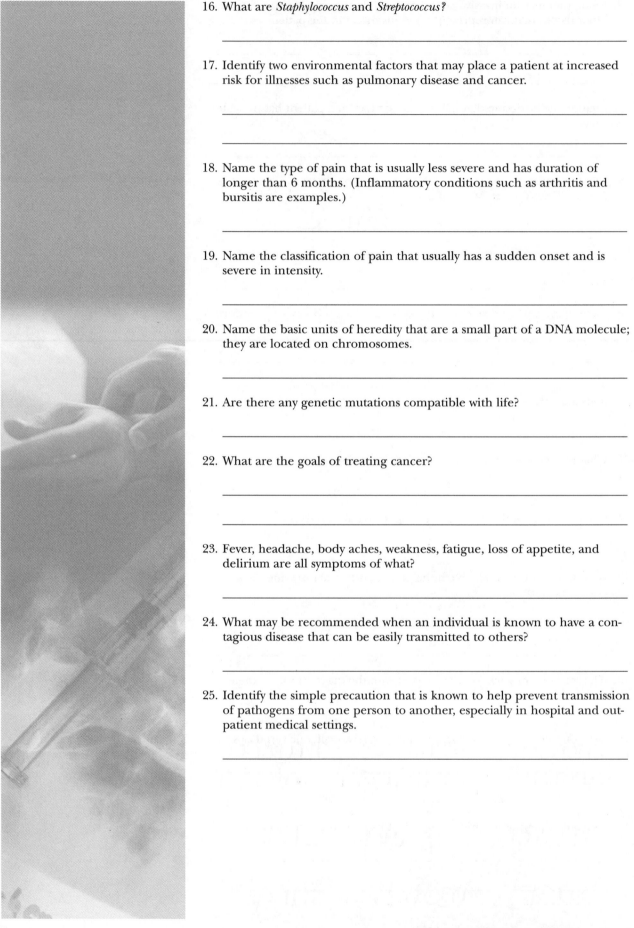

16. What are *Staphylococcus* and *Streptococcus?*

_____

17. Identify two environmental factors that may place a patient at increased risk for illnesses such as pulmonary disease and cancer.

_____

_____

18. Name the type of pain that is usually less severe and has duration of longer than 6 months. (Inflammatory conditions such as arthritis and bursitis are examples.)

_____

19. Name the classification of pain that usually has a sudden onset and is severe in intensity.

_____

20. Name the basic units of heredity that are a small part of a DNA molecule; they are located on chromosomes.

_____

21. Are there any genetic mutations compatible with life?

_____

22. What are the goals of treating cancer?

_____

_____

23. Fever, headache, body aches, weakness, fatigue, loss of appetite, and delirium are all symptoms of what?

_____

24. What may be recommended when an individual is known to have a contagious disease that can be easily transmitted to others?

_____

25. Identify the simple precaution that is known to help prevent transmission of pathogens from one person to another, especially in hospital and outpatient medical settings.

_____

Copyright ©2004, Elsevier. All rights reserved.

# FILL IN THE BLANKS

*Fill in the blanks with the correct terms. A Word List has been provided.*

1. Preventive health care emphasizes strategies for _____ a disease before it happens.

2. The X and Y chromosomes are known as ____Sex____ chromosomes.

3. Each person has ____23____ pairs of chromosomes. One chromosome from each pair is inherited from the ____father____ and one from the ____mother____.

4. The cardinal signs of infection include _____, _____, _____, _____, _____, _____, _____, and _____.

5. The ____CDC____ is a government agency responsible for publishing infectious disease reports in the United States after the diseases are reported to local health departments.

6. Tumors can be classified as either _____ or _____.

7. After evaluation, cancerous tissue is assigned a stage number ranging from I to IV, with stage ____I____ being an earlier stage tumor, which carries a better prognosis.

8. The _____ of cancer treatment is to eradicate every cancer cell in the body.

9. Chemotherapy involves the use of chemicals to eradicate cancer cells. The most common side effects are ____alopecia____, ____anorexia____, ____vomiting____, ____diarrhea____, ____anemia____, ____bruising____, and ____infertility____.

10. Physical trauma is the most common cause of death in ____children____ and ____young adults____.

11. A few examples of common allergens that are inhaled include ____dust____, ____molds____, and ____fungi____.

Copyright ©2004, Elsevier. All rights reserved.

12. When a person experiences pain, it is a warning sign that

_____ _____ is occurring.

13. Cultural diversity is recognized in the _____ realm of

medical treatment because health care providers must meet the needs of

culturally diverse patients.

14. Reflexology directs its efforts to the massage of the _____

and _____.

15. Genetic counseling is helpful in predicting _____ of

_____ of a gene-linked disease in a family.

## WORD LIST

I, 23, alopecia, anemia, anorexia, benign, bruising, Centers for Disease Control and Prevention (CDC), children, diarrhea, dust, enlarged lymph glands, father, feet, fever, fungi, goal, hands, heat, holistic, infertility, malignant, mold, mother, occurrence, pain, preventing, pus, redness, red streaks, risk, sex, swelling, tissue damage, vomiting, young adults

## ESSAY QUESTION

*Write a response to the following question or statement. Use a separate sheet of paper if more space is needed.*

Discuss the importance of recognizing cultural diversity in patients.

_____

_____

_____

_____

_____

_____

_____

_____

_____

_____

_____

_____

_____

_____

_____

Copyright ©2004, Elsevier. All rights reserved.

# CERTIFICATION EXAMINATION REVIEW

*Circle the letter of the choice that best completes the statement or answers the question.*

1. An abnormality in or mutation of a gene may produce which of the following?
   a. Inflammatory diseases
   b. Immunodeficiency disorders
   c. Genetic diseases
   d. None of the above

2. What types of tumors tend to metastasize and may spread to distant sites in the body?
   a. Malignant tumors
   b. Benign tumors
   c. Adipose tumors
   d. All of the above

3. Which of the following are included in the body's natural defense system against infection?
   a. Mechanical and chemical barriers
   b. Inflammatory response
   c. Immune response
   d. All of the above

4. Which of the following describe how a pathogen can cause disease?
   a. Intoxification
   b. Invasion and destruction of living tissue
   c. Infiltration of dead tissue
   d. Both a and b

5. Systemic manifestations of severe allergic responses include
   a. Itching
   b. Rash
   c. Anaphylaxis
   d. All of the above

6. The concept of medical care that focuses on the needs of the whole person—spiritual, cognitive, social, physical, and emotional—is the
   a. Holistic concept
   b. Hospice concept
   c. Osteopathy concept
   d. None of the above

7. The concept of care that affirms life and neither hastens or postpones death is the
   a. Holistic concept
   b. Hospice philosophy
   c. Osteopathy concept
   d. None of the above

8. Which of the following is responsible for stimulating the immune system to produce antibodies?
   a. Mutation
   b. Chromosome
   c. Antigen
   d. None of the above

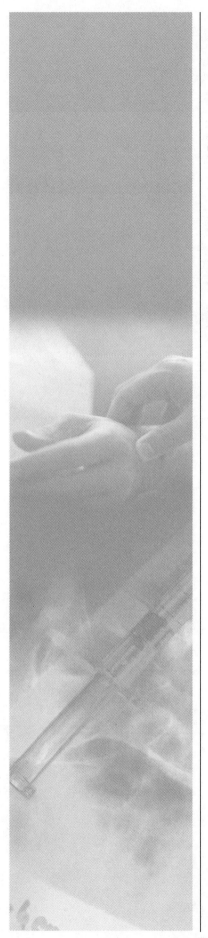

Copyright ©2004, Elsevier. All rights reserved.

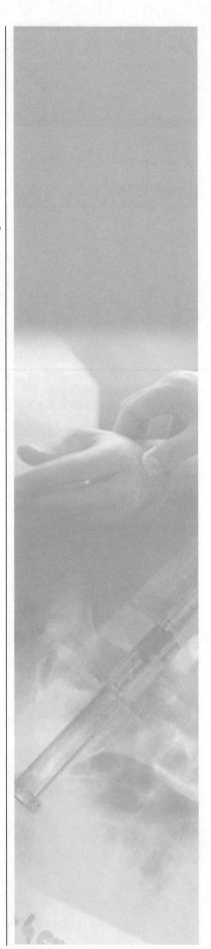

9. A new tissue growth or a tumor is called a
   a. Mutation
   b. Neoplasm
   c. Biopsy
   d. None of the above

10. Predisposing factors related to lifestyle include
    a. Gender
    b. Age
    c. Pollution of air and water
    d. Smoking, poor nutrition, lack of exercise, risky sexual behavior

Copyright ©2004, Elsevier. All rights reserved.

# CHAPTER 2

# Developmental, Congenital, and Childhood Diseases and Disorders

## WORD DEFINITIONS

*Define the following basic medical terms:*

1. Adduction _____

2. Apnea   *no breathing*

3. Arthritis   *inflamation of joints*

4. Bursitis   *inflamation of a bursa*

5. Congenital _____

6. Hydrocephalus _____

7. Hypovolemia   *lack of volume*

8. Lethargy   *sleepy; tired*

9. Myopia   *near sidedness*

10. Nosocomial   *infection related to*

11. Palpable   *to touch & diagnose*

12. Posterior   *pertaining to the back*

13. Postnatal   *after birth*

14. Postpartum   *after delivery*

15. Tracheostomy   *opening into the trachea*

16. Transdermal   *through the skin*

Copyright ©2004, Elsevier. All rights reserved.

# GLOSSARY TERMS

*Define the following chapter glossary terms:*

1. Anastomosis _____

2. Anorexia _____

3. Antipyretic _____

4. Cyanosis _____

5. Dysphagia _____

6. Dyspnea _____

7. Electromyography _____

8. Hemolysis _____

9. Hypertrophic _____

10. Hypoxia _____

11. Meconium _____

12. Necrosis _____

13. Normal flora _____

14. Photophobia _____

15. Phototherapy _____

16. Pruritus _____

17. Stenosis _____

18. Syncope _____

19. Tachycardia _____

20. Tachypnea _____

# SHORT ANSWER

*Answer the following questions:*

1. Can all congenital disorders be diagnosed by amniocentesis?

   _____

2. What occurs when there is a failure in the separation process of identical twins before the thirteenth day after fertilization?

   _____

3. The condition of conjoined twins is more prevalent in females or males?

   _____

Copyright ©2004, Elsevier. All rights reserved.

4. What is the weight range for premature infants?

_____

5. Name an example of an abnormality that may be detected by examination of amniotic fluid.

_____

6. What is another name for infant respiratory distress syndrome (IRDS)?

_____

7. Explain how retinopathy of prematurity (retrolental fibroplasias) is diagnosed.

_____

_____

8. Which is considered to be the most common crippling condition of children?

_____

9. Is the patient with cerebral palsy always mentally retarded?

_____

10. Identify the most serious form of spina bifida.

_____

11. If a baby is born with anencephaly, what is the prognosis?

_____

12. Name the most common congenital cardiac disorder.

_____

13. What color is the skin of a baby born with tetralogy of Fallot?

_____

14. Cite the statistics for the occurrence of cleft abnormalities.

_____

15. Name the most common kidney tumor of childhood.

_____

16. Is the cause of anemia the same in all cases?

_____

17. List examples of helminths that can live in the gastrointestinal (GI) tract.

_____

Copyright ©2004, Elsevier. All rights reserved.

18. Klinefelter syndrome and Turner syndrome are both chromosomal disorders. Which one affects males, and which one affects females?

_____

_____

19. The test for cystic fibrosis that measures the levels of sodium and chloride is called what?

_____

20. Identify the organism responsible for causing chicken pox.

_____

21. List a few precautions women can take to help decrease the risk of abnormal fetal development.

_____

_____

22. Cite possible causes of nongenetic congenital abnormalities that may be present in a child.

_____

23. List the three major types of cerebral palsy.

_____

_____

_____

24. Explain the goal of treatment for cerebral palsy.

_____

_____

25. List the four abnormalities present in the heart of an infant who has tetralogy of Fallot.

_____

_____

_____

_____

26. What are some of the physical characteristics that a child with Down syndrome will exhibit?

_____

_____

**12**

Copyright ©2004, Elsevier. All rights reserved.

27. Explain the treatment measures that may be used if clubfoot is present.

_____

_____

28. What treatment options are available to a baby born with patent ductus arteriosus (PDA)?

_____

_____

29. Define phimosis.

_____

30. List the symptoms associated with adenoid hyperplasia.

_____

31. What is the method of transmission for lead poisoning?

_____

# FILL IN THE BLANKS

*Fill in the blanks with the correct terms. A Word List has been provided.*

1. The diagnosis of congenital anomalies in a fetus can be accomplished by amniocentesis between the _____ and _____ week of pregnancy.

2. An infant with bronchopulmonary dysplasia (BPD) is very susceptible to respiratory infections such as _____ and _____.

3. Muscular dystrophy is diagnosed by _____ _____, _____, and _____ _____ _____ _____.

4. The exact cause of spina bifida is unknown. However, _____ and _____ factors may play a role. In addition, a decrease in the amount of _____ _____ and _____ _____ may contribute to the occurrence.

Copyright ©2004, Elsevier. All rights reserved.

5. Treatment for hydrocephalus usually includes placing a

_____ in the ventricular or subarachnoid spaces

to drain off the excessive cerebrospinal fluid (CSF).

6. An infant with cri du chat syndrome will exhibit an abnormally

_____ head, and if born alive, the infant will

have a weak _____, catlike cry.

7. Congenital _____ defects are developmental

anomalies of the heart or _____

_____ of the heart.

8. An atrial septic defect that is large would cause pronounced symptoms of

_____, _____, and

_____.

9. The prognosis for cleft lip and cleft palate is _____

with surgical repair.

10. An infant with _____ _____

has episodes of projectile vomiting after feedings. The onset of symptoms

usually begins within 2 to 3 weeks after birth.

11. Phenylketonuria is an inborn error in the metabolism of amino acids

that causes _____ _____ and

_____ _____ if not treated.

12. Diphtheria can be prevented by the administration of

_____ _____ to produce active immunity.

13. The causative agent of mumps is an _____ virus, which

is spread by _____ nuclei from the respiratory tract.

14. The drug of choice to treat pertussis (whooping cough) is

_____.

15. The incubation period for tetanus is _____ to _____ days, with the

onset commonly occurring at about _____ days.

## WORD LIST

3, 8, 21, fifteenth, eighteenth, airborne, brain damage, cardiac, cyanosis, diphtheria toxoid, droplet, dyspnea, electromyography (EMG), elevated serum creatinine kinase (CK), environmental, erythromycin, folic acid, genetic, good, great vessels, mental retardation, mewing, muscle biopsy, pneumonia, pyloric stenosis, RSV, shunt, small, syncope, vitamin A

Copyright ©2004, Elsevier. All rights reserved.

# ANATOMIC STRUCTURES

*Label the following anatomic diagrams. For number 2, identify the correct heart defect that each diagram illustrates.*

1. Circulation patterns before and after birth

## Fetal Circulation

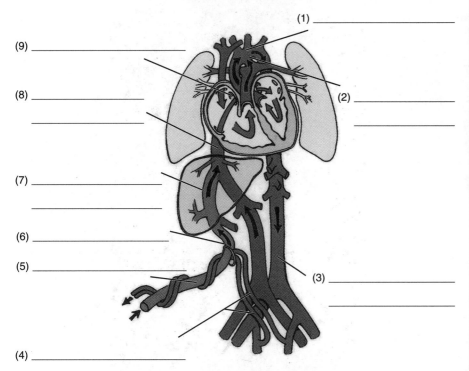

(1) _____

(9) _____

(8) _____

_____

(2) _____

_____

(7) _____

_____

(6) _____

(5) _____

(3) _____

_____

(4) _____

## Circulation after Birth

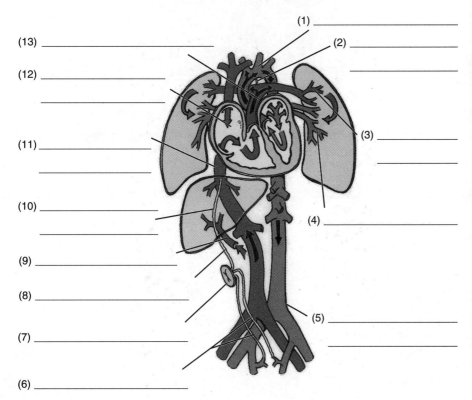

(1) _____

(13) _____

(2) _____

(12) _____

_____

(11) _____

(3) _____

_____

(10) _____

(4) _____

(9) _____

(8) _____

(5) _____

(7) _____

_____

(6) _____

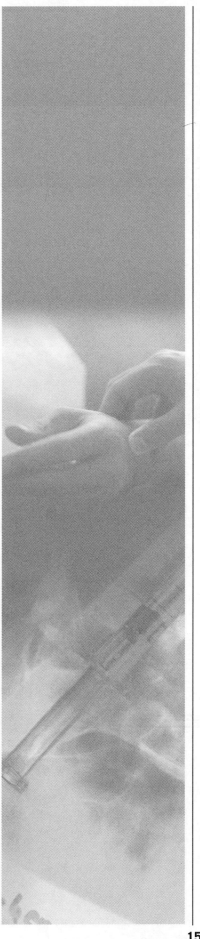

Copyright ©2004, Elsevier. All rights reserved.

2. Heart defects

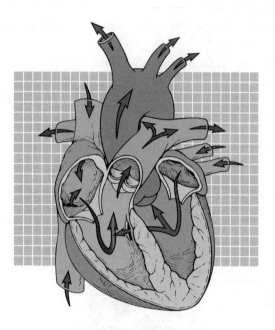

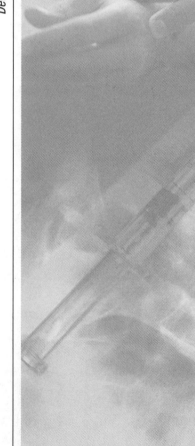

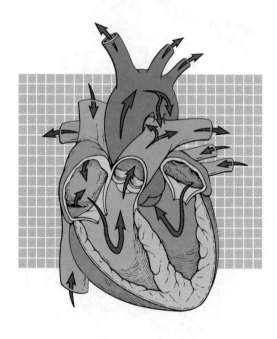

Copyright ©2004, Elsevier. All rights reserved.

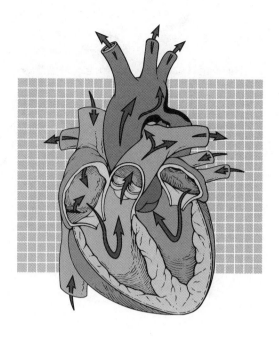

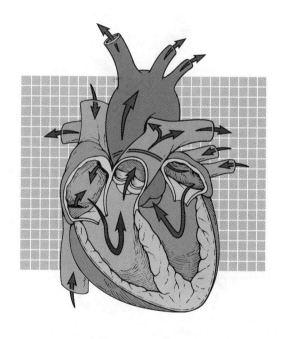

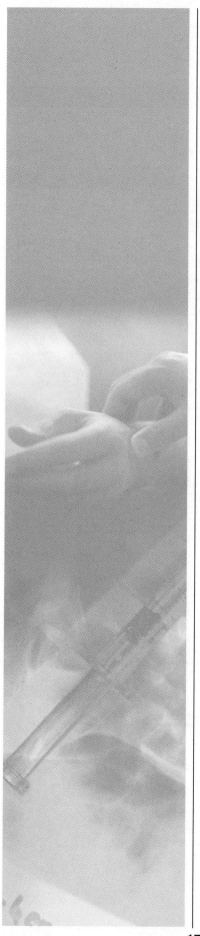

Copyright ©2004, Elsevier. All rights reserved.

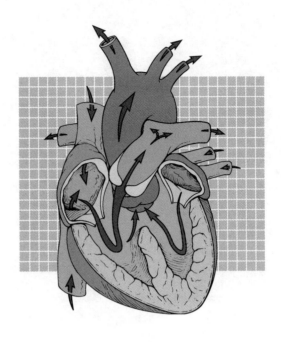

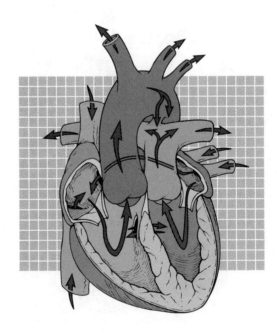

Transportation of the Great Arteries

Copyright ©2004, Elsevier. All rights reserved.

# PATIENT SCREENING

*For each scenario that follows, explain how and why you would schedule an appointment or suggest a referral based on the patient's reported symptoms.* **First, review the "Guidelines for Patient-Screening Exercises" found on page iv in the "Introduction."**

1. The mother of a 6-month-old infant calls the office requesting an appointment for her child. She advises that she thinks the child's head appears swollen and that there are areas that appear to be bulging. What is your response regarding the appointment?

   _____

   _____

   _____

2. The mother of a 3-year-old boy calls to report her child had the onset of vomiting and abdominal pain during the night and is now experiencing blood in his urine. She says she just noticed a swelling on his left side toward his back. She requests an appointment. What is your response regarding the appointment?

   _____

   _____

   _____

3. The mother of a 15-day-old infant son reports that he started having episodes of vomiting with the emesis "shooting out of his mouth" after feeding. She also reports the infant appears hungry, continues to feed, and has not gained any weight. How do you respond to this phone call?

   _____

   _____

   _____

4. Just as the office is closing for the day, a mother calls about her child who just started experiencing signs and symptoms of respiratory distress including hoarseness; fever; a harsh, high-pitched cough; and a funny, high-pitched sound during inspiration. The physician has already left the office for the day. How do you handle this call?

   _____

   _____

   _____

5. A mother calls to report that her three children have been complaining of being fatigued, having headaches, and stomach, muscle, and joint pain for the past 2 weeks. She also states there has been a significant change in their behavior. How do you handle this call?

   _____

   _____

   _____

Copyright ©2004, Elsevier. All rights reserved.

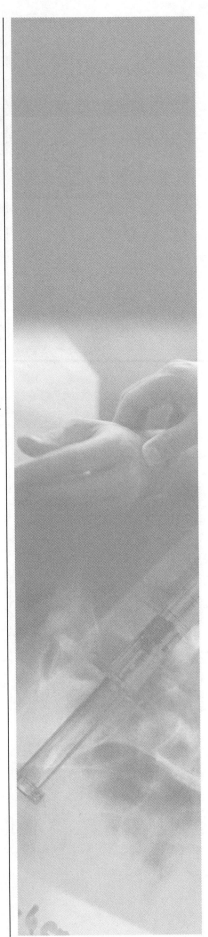

# PATIENT TEACHING

*For each scenario that follows, outline the appropriate patient teaching you would per-*
*form.* **First, review the "Guidelines for Patient-Teaching Exercises" found on page iv**
**in the "Introduction."**

1. **SPINA BIFIDA**
   Parents have brought the previously diagnosed child to the office for a
   routine visit. They missed the last regularly scheduled appointment.
   During the intake assessment, they told you the child had no problems
   so they just did not come. How do you handle this patient
   (parent)–teaching opportunity?

   _____

   _____

   _____

   _____

2. **PYLORIC STENOSIS**
   An infant has been seen on its first postoperative follow-up visit. How do
   you handle this patient (parent)–teaching opportunity?

   _____

   _____

   _____

   _____

3. **CHICKEN POX**
   A child has just been diagnosed with chicken pox. How do you handle
   this patient (parent)–teaching opportunity?

   _____

   _____

   _____

   _____

4. **TONSILLITIS**
   A child has just been diagnosed with tonsillitis. The physician has prescribed a round of antibiotics for the child. He has also made note to the
   parents to ensure that the child has adequate hydration. How do you
   handle this patient (parent)–teaching opportunity?

   _____

   _____

   _____

   _____

Copyright ©2004, Elsevier. All rights reserved.

5. **ASTHMA**

A child has been examined for a severe episode of recurring asthma. The physician has prescribed a prophylactic inhalant to be used before exposure. In addition, the child has a prescription for a bronchodilator medication that he is inconsistent in taking. How do you handle this patient (parent)–teaching opportunity?

_____

_____

_____

_____

## ESSAY QUESTION

*Write a response to the following question or statement. Use a separate sheet of paper if more space is needed.*

Compare the symptoms of the three major types of cerebral palsy: spastic cerebral palsy, athetoid cerebral palsy, and ataxic cerebral palsy.

_____

_____

_____

_____

_____

_____

_____

## CERTIFICATION EXAMINATION REVIEW

*Circle the letter of the choice that best completes the statement or answers the question.*

1. Reye syndrome has been associated with the use of
   a. Acetaminophen.
   b. Ibuprofen.
   c. Aspirin.
   d. All of the above.

2. Loss of appetite, vomiting, irritability, and ataxic gait are symptoms associated with
   a. Muscular dystrophy.
   b. Anemia.
   c. Lead poisoning.
   d. All of the above.

3. The leading cause of absenteeism in school children is
   a. Asthma.
   b. Strep infections.
   c. Bronchitis.
   d. None of the above.

Copyright ©2004, Elsevier. All rights reserved.

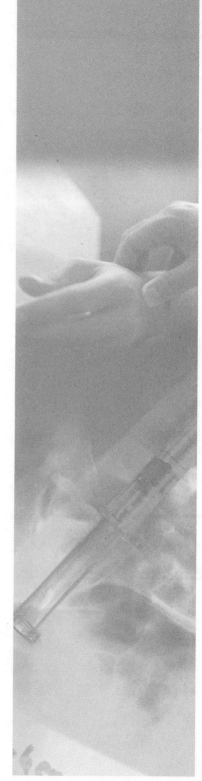

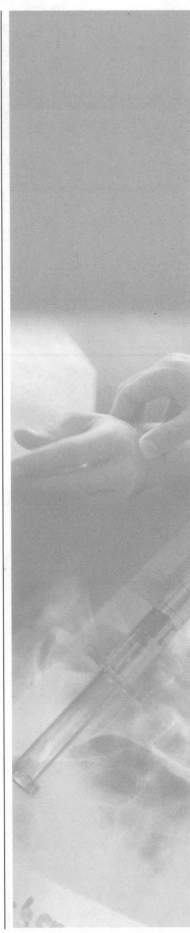

4. The failure of the testicle(s) to descend into the scrotum is called
   a. Cryptorchidism.
   b. Testicular torsion.
   c. Phimosis.
   d. None of the above.

5. If a child is born with tetralogy of Fallot, how many actual heart defects are present?
   a. Two
   b. Three
   c. Four
   d. None of the above

6. When a person is diagnosed with leukemia, there will be a/an
   a. Increase in white blood cells.
   b. Decrease in white blood cells.
   c. Normal white blood cell count.
   d. None of the above.

7. A sensitivity to iron or cow's milk may cause
   a. Cystic fibrosis.
   b. Infantile colic.
   c. Pyloric stenosis.
   d. All of the above.

8. The most progressive form of muscular dystrophy is
   a. Occulta.
   b. Duchenne.
   c. Down.
   d. None of the above.

9. One method of preventing epidemics of contagious diseases is to administer
   a. Aspirin.
   b. Immunizations.
   c. Multivitamins.
   d. None of the above.

10. Hypertension, hematuria, and pain are symptoms of
    a. Leukemia.
    b. Cystic fibrosis.
    c. Wilms tumor.
    d. All of the above.

11. The number one cause of death in children between the ages of 1 month and 1 year is
    a. Sudden infant death syndrome.
    b. Cystic fibrosis.
    c. Down syndrome.
    d. Erythroblastosis fetalis.

12. Rheumatic fever, kidney complications, and rheumatic heart disease may be complications of untreated
    a. Lead poisoning.
    b. Tonsillitis caused by A beta-hemolytic streptococci.
    c. Vomiting and diarrhea.
    d. None of the above.

13. Intracranial pressure is present when cerebrospinal fluid accumulates in the skull when the patient has
    a. Hydrocephalus.
    b. Spina bifida.
    c. Fetal alcohol syndrome.
    d. None of the above.

Copyright ©2004, Elsevier. All rights reserved.

# CHAPTER 3

# Immunologic Diseases and Conditions

## WORD DEFINITIONS

*Define the following basic medical terms:*

1. Allograft — a homograft between allogenic individuals

2. Arthralgia — pain in one or more joints

3. Conjunctivitis — inflamation of the conjunctiva

4. Ecchymosis — escape of blood into the tissues from ruptured blood vessels by a livid black/blue spot/area.

5. Endocrinopathies — disease marked by dysfunction of an endocrine gland

6. Exacerbate — to cause a disease to become more severe

7. Flatulence — quality/state of being flatulent

8. Hypocalcemia — deficiency of calcium in the blood

9. Lysis — gradual decline of a disease process (as fever)

10. Neuritis — inflammatory lesion of a nerve marked esp. by pain or lost reflexes

11. Ocular — of or relating to the eye

12. Splenomegaly — abnormal enlargement of the spleen

13. Spondylitis — inflamation of the vertebrae

14. Stomatitis — inflammatory disease of the mouth

15. Thyroiditis — inflamation of the thyroid gland

16. Uveitis — inflamation of the uvea

17. Vasculitis — inflamation of a blood or lymph vessel

Copyright ©2004, Elsevier. All rights reserved.

# GLOSSARY TERMS

*Define the following chapter glossary terms:*

1. Antibodies — immunoglobulin that may combine with a specific antigen to destroy or control it

2. Antigens — any substance that stimulates the immune system to produce antibodies

3. Atrophy — wasting away; tissue, cell or organ

4. Autoimmune — immune response is misdirected

5. Discoid — shaped like a disk

6. Enzyme-linked immunosorbent assay — test used to detect antibodies of AIDS virus in the blood stream

7. Erythrocyte sedimentation rate (ESR) — measurable reflection of acute-phase reaction in inflammation and infection

8. Idiopathic — refers to a disease without a known or recognizable cause

9. Immunocompetence — the ability of the immune system to defend the body against disease

10. Immunodeficiency — inability to produce a normal complement of antibodies

11. Immunoglobulins — protein that can act as an antibody

12. Immunosuppressive — property of suppressing the body's immune response to antigens

13. Ischemic — holding back / obstructing blood flow

14. Macrophages — monocyte blood cell

15. Megakaryocytes — large bone marrow cell having large or many nuclei

16. Megaloblastic — pertaining to abnormally large RBC's found in pernicious anemia

17. Opportunistic infections — infection resulting from a defective immune system

18. Petechiae — tiny spider like hemorrhage under the skin

19. Phagocytes — process by which cells surround and digest certain particles

20. Phagocytosis — Same as #19

21. Reticuloendothelial — 

22. Retrovirus — 

23. Tetany — 

24. Thrombocytopenia — reduced number of thrombocytes

25. Western blot test — 

Copyright ©2004, Elsevier. All rights reserved.

# SHORT ANSWER

*Answer the following questions:*

1. What would be included as primary lymphoid tissues?

   _____

2. Which structures are considered the first line of defense against foreign substances or antigens?

   _____

3. How many types of immunity are there, and what are they called?

   _____

   _____

4. What is the name of the substance that coats B cells, providing them with the ability to recognize foreign protein, stimulating the antigen-antibody reaction?

   _____

5. What is the name of the virus that causes acquired immunodeficiency syndrome (AIDS)?

   *human immunodeficiency virus (HIV)*

6. Identify the organism responsible for causing a fungal infection of the mucous membranes of the mouth, genitalia, or skin. It is a common opportunistic infection observed in patients who have AIDS.

   *candida albicans; yes*

7. Is there a cure for AIDS?

   *no there is not*

8. Severe combined immunodeficiency (SCID) results from disturbances in the development and function of what cells?

   *T cells and B cells t*

9. Identify the treatment option for SCID.

   *bone marrow transplantation*

10. When a patient has autoimmune hemolytic anemia, antibodies destroy what?

    *red blood cells*

11. What is the last treatment used for thrombocytopenic purpura?

    _____

    _____

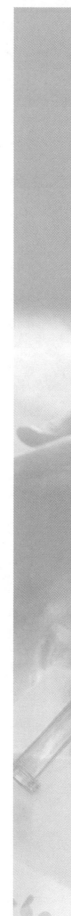

Copyright ©2004, Elsevier. All rights reserved.

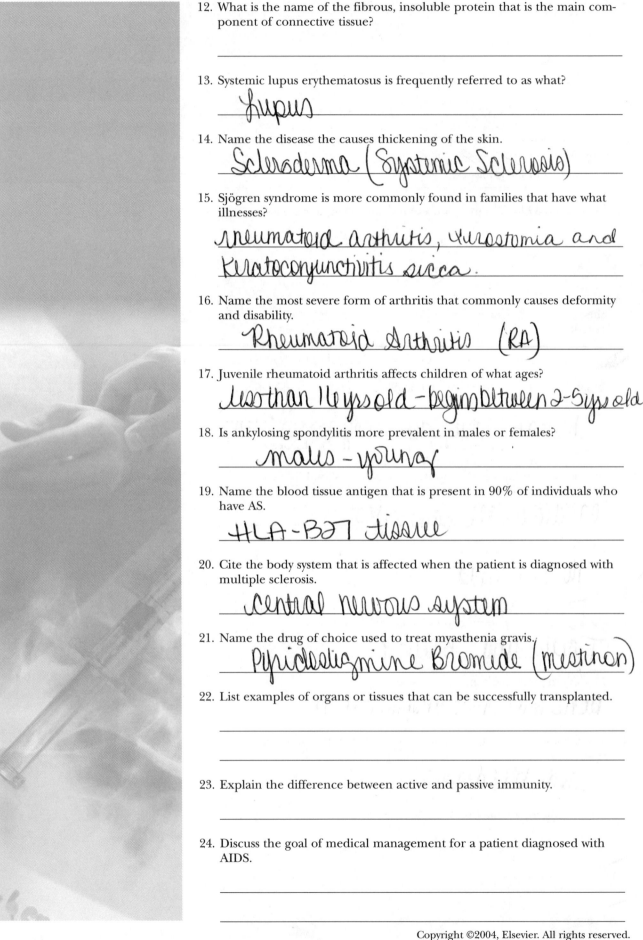

12. What is the name of the fibrous, insoluble protein that is the main component of connective tissue?

_____

13. Systemic lupus erythematosus is frequently referred to as what?

*Lupus*

14. Name the disease the causes thickening of the skin.

*Scleroderma (Systemic Sclerosis)*

15. Sjögren syndrome is more commonly found in families that have what illnesses?

*rheumatoid arthritis, xerostomia and Keratoconjunctivitis sicca.*

16. Name the most severe form of arthritis that commonly causes deformity and disability.

*Rheumatoid Arthritis (RA)*

17. Juvenile rheumatoid arthritis affects children of what ages?

*less than 16 yrs old - begins between 2-5 yrs old*

18. Is ankylosing spondylitis more prevalent in males or females?

*males - young*

19. Name the blood tissue antigen that is present in 90% of individuals who have AS.

*HLA-B27 tissue*

20. Cite the body system that is affected when the patient is diagnosed with multiple sclerosis.

*Central nervous system*

21. Name the drug of choice used to treat myasthenia gravis.

*Pyridostigmine Bromide (mestinon)*

22. List examples of organs or tissues that can be successfully transplanted.

_____

_____

23. Explain the difference between active and passive immunity.

_____

24. Discuss the goal of medical management for a patient diagnosed with AIDS.

_____

_____

Copyright ©2004, Elsevier. All rights reserved.

25. Explain the precautions for immunizing children with Bruton's agamma-globulinemia.

_____

_____

## FILL IN THE BLANKS

*Fill in the blanks with the correct terms. A Word List has been provided. Words used twice are indicated with a (2).*

1. The __immune__ __system__ is responsible for a complex response to the invasion of the body by foreign substances.

2. Macrophages, which develop from __monocytes__, are found in the tissues of the liver, lungs, or lymph nodes.

3. If a patient has a positive enzyme-linked immunosorbent assay (ELISA) for human immunodeficiency viral (HIV) antibodies, the tests should be confirmed with another test called a __western__ __blot__.

4. Common variable immunodeficiency is an acquired __B__ __cell__ __deficiency__ that results in an absence of antibody production or function or both.

5. DiGeorge anomaly is identified in children who have structural anomalies such as wide-set, downward slanting __eyes__, low-set ears with notched __pinnas__, a small __mouth__, and __cardiovascular__ defects.

6. The drug of choice to treat chronic mucocutaneous candidiasis is __mycostatin__.

7. The child who has the diagnosis of Wiskott-Aldrich syndrome experiences __thrombocytopenia__ and eczema.

8. Autoimmune diseases occur when __autoantibodies__ develop and begin to destroy the body's own __cells__.

9. Symptoms associated with pernicious anemia include a __sore__ __tongue__, __weakness__, __tingling__, and __numbness__ in the extremities. They may also have disturbances in digestion as a result of a decrease in the production of __hydrochloric__ __acid__.

Copyright ©2004, Elsevier. All rights reserved.

10. Monthly injections of __vitamin_____ B₁₂__ are used to treat pernicious anemia.

11. The cause of thrombocytopenic purpura is often considered __idiopathic__ although antibodies that reduce the life of __platelets__ have been found in most cases.

12. Symptoms of Goodpasture syndrome are __acute__ __glomerulonephritis__, relatively acute __renal__ __failure__ with __proteinuria__, anemia hemoptysis, and __hematuria__.

13. Treatment options for collagen diseases are directed at quieting the over-active __immune__ __system__.

14. The primary objectives of treatment for rheumatoid arthritis are the __reduction__ of __inflammation__ and pain, preservation of joint __function__, and the prevention of joint __deformity__.

15. The __spinal__ __column__ is usually affected by ankylosing spondylitis.

16. The most common symptom of polymyositis is __weakness__ of the __muscles__.

17. Prolonged exposure to __sunlight__, __cold__, __infections__ and emotional __stress__ exacerbate the symptoms of myasthenia gravis.

## WORD LIST

acute glomerulonephritis, autoantibodies, B cell deficiency, cardiovascular, cells, deformity, eyes, function, hematuria, hydrochloric acid, idiopathic, immune system (2), infections, inflammation, monocytes, mouth, muscles, mycostatin, numbness, pinnas, platelets, proteinuria, reduction, renal failure, sore tongue, spinal column, stress, sunlight, thrombocytopenia, tingling, vitamin B12, weakness (2), western blot

Copyright ©2004, Elsevier. All rights reserved.

# ANATOMIC STRUCTURES

*Identify the following structures of the immune system.*

1. Immune system

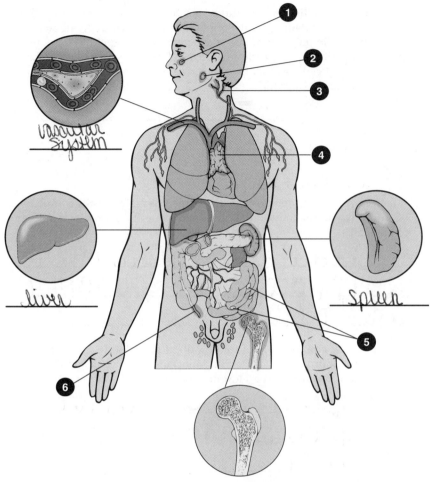

vascular system

liver

spleen

bone marrow

(1) __adenoids__     (4) __thymus gland__

(2) __tonsil__     (5) __peyer patches of small intestine__

(3) __lymph node__     (6) __appendix__

Copyright ©2004, Elsevier. All rights reserved.

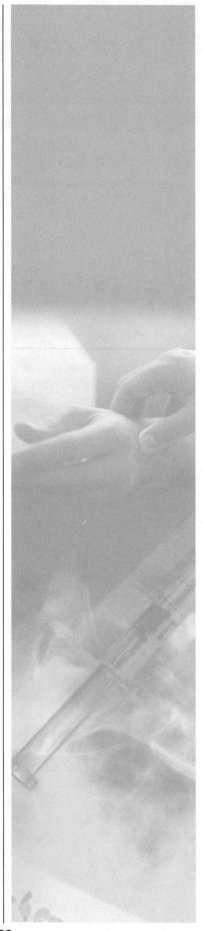

# PATIENT SCREENING

*For each scenario below, explain how and why you would schedule an appointment or suggest a referral based on the patient's reported symptoms.* **First, review the "Guidelines for Patient-Screening Exercises" found on page iv in the "Introduction."**

1. A woman calls to discuss a condition her husband is experiencing. She reports he is complaining of feeling fatigued and experiencing weakness. Additionally, she tells you he has started experiencing chills, has a fever, and is complaining of shortness of breath. She also states that his skin is pale and jaundiced and that he appears to bruise easily. How do you respond to this phone call?

_____

_____

_____

2. A patient previously diagnosed with pernicious anemia calls complaining of an increased weakness and a rapid heart rate. How do you handle this phone call?

*schedule an apuntnmut so the doctor can prescribe any medications*

3. A patient calls complaining of spitting up blood, blood in his urine, and a reduced amount of urine. He also mentions a recent weight loss, being fatigued, and having a fever. How do you handle this phone call?

*tell him should see the doctor asap or be admitted to the hospital*

4. The female patient calls stating she is experiencing an unexplained weight loss, fatigue, a persistent low-grade fever, and general malaise. She also mentions joint stiffness, especially on wakening and during periods of inactivity. She is requesting an appointment for an evaluation and treatment of her symptoms. How do you respond to her?

_____

_____

_____

5. A patient has previously been diagnosed with polymyositis. This patient calls the office complaining of a sudden significant loss of strength and some problems swallowing. How do you handle this phone call?

_____

_____

_____

Copyright ©2004, Elsevier. All rights reserved.

# PATIENT TEACHING

*For each scenario below, outline the appropriate patient teaching you would perform.*
**First, review the "Guidelines for Patient-Teaching Exercises" found on page iv in the**
**"Introduction."**

1. **COMMON VARIABLE IMMUNODEFICIENCY (ACQUIRED) HYPOGAMMAGLOBULINEMIA**
   Diagnosis of common variable immunodeficiency (acquired) hypogamma-globulinemia has just been confirmed. The physician has printed information for patients about this disorder. How do you handle this patient-teaching opportunity?

   _____

   _____

   _____

2. **CHRONIC MUCOCUTANEOUS CANDIDIASIS**
   A diagnosis of chronic mucocutaneous candidiasis has just been confirmed. The physician has printed material concerning this disorder. You have been instructed to provide this information to the patient and to discuss comfort measures for mouth care. How do you handle this patient-teaching opportunity?

   _____

   _____

   _____

3. **IDIOPATHIC THROMBOCYTOPENIC PURPURA**
   The child has been diagnosed with idiopathic thrombocytopenic purpura, and infusion therapy is probably going to be prescribed. The physician has printed information regarding this therapy and treatment of this disorder. You are instructed to use this printed information and to discuss it with the family. How do you handle this patient-teaching opportunity?

   _____

   _____

   _____

4. **RHEUMATOID ARTHRITIS**
   A patient with rheumatoid arthritis has just concluded a visit with the physician. The physician has printed material concerning the cause and treatment options for this disorder. You have been instructed to discuss this material with the patient. How do you handle this patient-teaching opportunity?

   _____

   _____

   _____

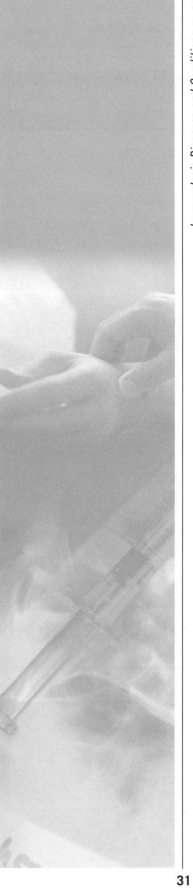

Copyright ©2004, Elsevier. All rights reserved.

5. **MULTIPLE SCLEROSIS**

A patient with multiple sclerosis has experienced an exacerbation of the condition. The physician has printed materials regarding possible treatments of and medications prescribed for this disorder. You are instructed to review this material with the patient. How do you handle this patient-teaching opportunity?

_____

_____

_____

## ESSAY QUESTION

_Write a response to the following question or statement. Use a separate sheet of paper if more space is needed._

Discuss the guidelines that are included in infection control and Universal Precautions and their importance in the safety of the health care worker.

_____

_____

_____

_____

_____

_____

_____

_____

_____

_____

_____

_____

_____

_____

_____

_____

_____

_____

Copyright ©2004, Elsevier. All rights reserved.

# CERTIFICATION EXAMINATION REVIEW

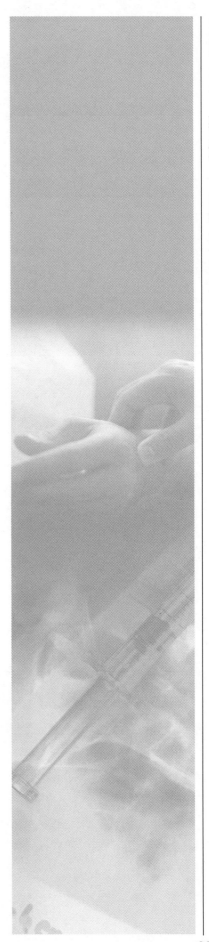

*Circle the letter of the choice that best completes the statement or answers the question.*

1. Idiopathic thrombocytopenic anemia involves a deficiency of platelets and
   a. A decrease in red blood cell count
   b. A decrease in white blood cell count
   c. The inability of blood to clot
   d. None of the above

2. Active immunity is acquired when a person
   a. Has a disease
   b. Receives an immunization
   c. Is born
   d. None of the above

3. Autoimmune diseases occur when
   a. A person's immune system reacts appropriately to an antigen and homeostasis is maintained.
   b. Antibodies develop and begin to destroy the body's own cells.
   c. A person fails to receive childhood immunizations.
   d. All of the above are true.

4. Symptoms of butterfly rash, fever, joint pain, malaise, and weight loss are present with
   a. Scleroderma
   b. Systemic lupus erythematosus
   c. Rheumatoid arthritis
   d. None of the above

5. Symptoms of inflammation and edema are present at the onset of
   a. Scleroderma
   b. Systemic lupus erythematosus
   c. Rheumatoid arthritis
   d. None of the above

6. Symptoms of hardening and shrinking of the skin are associated with
   a. Scleroderma
   b. Systemic lupus erythematosus
   c. Rheumatoid arthritis
   d. None of the above

7. Myasthenia gravis is treated with
   a. Mestinon
   b. Vitamin B12
   c. Both a and b
   d. None of the above

8. The thymus glands produce
   a. A-cell lymphocytes
   b. C-cell lymphocytes
   c. T-cell lymphocytes
   d. All of the above

9. HIV is transmitted by
   a. Close physical contact
   b. Blood and body fluids
   c. Both a and b
   d. None of the above

Copyright ©2004, Elsevier. All rights reserved.

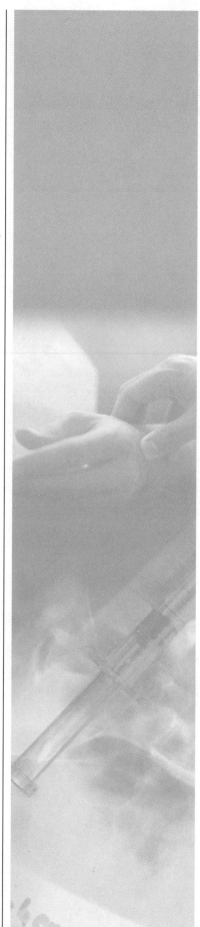

10. Selective immunoglobulin A deficiency disease is
    a. The most common form of immunodeficiency
    b. The least common form of immunodeficiency
    c. Transmitted by close casual contact
    d. None of the above

11. Pernicious anemia is treated with
    a. Blood transfusions
    b. Vitamin B12
    c. Plasma
    d. None of the above

12. Ankylosing spondyliasis primarily affects the
    a. Shoulder
    b. Spine
    c. Knee
    d. All of the above

13. Multiple sclerosis is an inflammatory disease that attacks
    a. The joints
    b. The spinal nerves
    c. The myelin sheath
    d. None of the above

14. Myasthenia gravis is a chronic progressive disease that is characterized by
    a. Muscle stiffness
    b. Extreme muscular weakness and progressive fatigue
    c. Pain
    d. None of the above

Copyright ©2004, Elsevier. All rights reserved.

# CHAPTER 4

# Diseases and Conditions of the Endocrine System

## WORD DEFINITIONS

*Define the following basic medical terms:*

1. Anterior — front of the body
2. Atrophy — decrease in size
3. Copious —
4. Dysfunction — abnormal function
5. Encephalopathy — disease of the brain
6. Fatigue — exhaustion from labor
7. Flatus — gas generated in the stomach or bowel
8. Hyperplasia —
9. Hyposecretion — bodily secretion production @ a slow rate
10. Hypotension — abnormally low BP
11. Inspection — visual observation of the body during a physical examination
12. Palpation — act of touching or feeling during examination
13. Palpitation — rapid pulsation
14. Polydipsia — excessive thirst
15. Polyphagia — excessive eating
16. Polyuria — excessive urination
17. Specific gravity —
18. Tremor — trembling or shaking
19. Turgor — normal state of turgidity and tension in living cells

Copyright ©2004, Elsevier. All rights reserved.

# GLOSSARY TERMS

*Define the following chapter glossary terms:*

1. Adenoma — a benign tumor of a glandular structure

2. Corticotropin — hormone secreted by the anterior lobe of the pituitary

3. Dysphagia — difficulty swallowing

4. Endemic — disease or condition found in a certain population/region

5. Epiphyseal — ends of the bone where bone growth occurs

6. Goitrogenic — pertaining to substances causing goiters

7. Hyperglycemia — increase in blood glucose level

8. Hyperlipidemia — increase in fat levels in blood

9. Hyperparathyroidism — condition caused by overactive parathyroid gland

10. Hypertrophy — enlargement of any organ/structure

11. Idiopathic — refers to a disease without a known cause

12. Infarct — area of dead blood tissue caused by lack of blood supply

13. Metastasize — spreading of the disease from 1 part to another not directly connected

14. Panhypopituitarism — entire pituitary gland not functioning

15. Pathogenesis — development of a disease

16. Pruritus — itching

17. Radioimmunoassay — test that measures minute amounts of antibodies by radioactive substances

18. Stridor — high-pitched respiratory sound caused by obstruction in air passages

19. Sulfonylureas — oral hypoglycemic agent that stimulates the pancreas to produce insulin

20. Syncope — fainting; lightheadedness

# SHORT ANSWER

*Answer the following questions:*

1. Name the master gland of the endocrine system.

2. Identify the hormones responsible for stimulating secretion of other hormones.

    endocrine — topic

3. Endocrine diseases result from an abnormal secretion of what?

    increase or decrease in the secretion of hormones

Copyright ©2004, Elsevier. All rights reserved.

4. Name three types of laboratory tests that may be used to evaluate hormone levels.

_____

5. Acromegaly and gigantism are conditions resulting from an overproduction of which hormone?

_____*pituitary hormones*_____

6. Identify the term used for the abnormal underdevelopment of the body occurring in children.

_____*dwarfism*_____

7. Diabetes insipidus is more common in males or females?

_____*males*_____

8. Name the most common endocrine gland to produce a disease condition or problem.

_____

9. Identify the hormone released from the pituitary gland that controls the activity of the thyroid gland.

_____

10. Is Hashimoto disease more common in male or female patients? Cite statistics of incidence in comparing the sexes.

_____*females; women 8 times as often as in men*_____

11. Describe the most outstanding clinical feature of Hashimoto disease.

_____*enlargement of the thyroid gland*_____

12. Name the branch of medicine that deals with endocrine disorders.

_____

13. List two examples of ways to ensure ingestion of iodine.

_____

14. Describe the goal of treatment for a patient with Graves disease.

_____

15. Cite the age range during which cretinism develops.

_____*infancy or early childhood*_____

16. Name the therapeutic agent that is administered to treat myxedema.

_____*Levothyroxine Sodium (T4)*_____

17. List the four main types of thyroid cancer.

_____*papillary, follicular, medullary, anaplastic*_____

Copyright ©2004, Elsevier. All rights reserved.

18. Of the four types, identify the most common type of thyroid cancer.

_papillary and follicular_

19. Describe the symptoms of Cushing syndrome.

_they experience fatigue, muscular weakness and changes in body appearance_

20. Explain the treatment for Addison disease.

_increase a fluid, control of salt,_

21. List five oral medications that are commonly used to treat type 2 diabetes.

_glipizide (Glucotrol), glyburide (Diabeta or Micronase), Glucophage, Precose, Actos & Avandia_

22. Name the organs that can be damaged if blood glucose levels are not controlled.

23. Identify the type of diabetes that has its onset during pregnancy.

_gestational Diabetes_

24. Cite the numbers associated with abnormally low levels of plasma glucose in women and men after a period of fasting.

25. At what age is puberty considered precocious in male adolescents?

_before 9 years old_

26. At what age is puberty considered precocious in female adolescents?

_before 8 years old_

27. Identify the hormone responsible for promoting bone and tissue growth.

28. Identify the hormone responsible for regulating skin pigmentation.

29. Name the hormone that causes uterine contractions.

30. Name the hormone that causes development of female secondary sex characteristics.

Copyright ©2004, Elsevier. All rights reserved.

# FILL IN THE BLANKS

*Fill in the blanks with the correct terms. A Word List has been provided.*

1. The action of most hormones is directed to target _glands_ or _tissues_ at distant receptor sites, thereby regulating critical body functions such as _urinary output_, cellular metabolic rate, and _growth_ and _development_.

2. A frequent cause of an over-secretion of human growth hormone (hGH) is an _anterior pituitary adenoma_.

3. The cause of hypopituitarism may be a _pituitary_ tumor or a tumor of the _hypothalamus_. Some causes are _congenital_ deficiencies. It may also be the result of damage to the _pituitary_ gland.

4. The treatment for dwarfism is the administration of _somatotropin (hgh)_ until the child reaches the height of 5 feet.

5. Two symptoms of diabetes insipidus are _extreme thirst_ and secretion of _dilute urine_.

6. A _goiter_ is often the first sign of thyroid disease.

7. The two hormones produced by the thyroid gland are _thyroxine (T4)_ and _tri-iodothyronine (T3)_.

8. The cause of Hashimoto disease is unknown, but a _genetic factor_ is suggested.

9. A patient with Graves disease exhibits symptoms of _rapid heartbeat_, _palpitations_, nervousness, _excitability_ and _insomnia_. There may be other symptoms present in addition to these.

10. A child with cretinism may have symptoms that include _mental_ and _growth_ retardation.

11. The face of the patient with _myxedema_ becomes bloated, the tongue _thick_, and the eyelids _puffy_.

Copyright ©2004, Elsevier. All rights reserved.

12. Thyroid tumors that are undifferentiated, rare, and occur mainly in patients over 60 years of age are _anaplastic_

13. Hyperparathyroidism increases the _breakdown_ of _bone_ with the subsequent release of _excessive calcium_ and extracellular fluid.

14. The patient with Addison disease would exhibit elevated serum _potassium_, blood urea nitrogen, _lymphocyte_ and eosinophil levels, and elevated _hematocrit_

15. Patients with type _II_ diabetes do not usually require insulin to control blood glucose levels.

16. Thirty to _40_ percent of women who have had gestational diabetes mellitus (GDM) develop type 2 diabetes within 5 to 10 years after giving birth.

17. An individual with severe symptoms of _acute reactive_ hypoglycemia requires _emergency_ medical attention.

18. Precocious puberty in the male adolescent is exhibited by early development of _secondary sex_ characteristics, _gonadal_ development, and spermatogenesis.

19. In most cases the cause of precocious puberty in females is _idiopathic_ without associated abnormalities.

20. The hormone responsible for initiating growth of eggs in the ovaries and simulating spermatogenesis in the testes is called _follicle stimulating hormone_.

## WORD LIST

II, acute reactive, anaplastic, anterior pituitary adenoma, bone, breakdown, congenital, damage, dilute urine, emergency, excessive calcium, excitability, extreme thirst, follicle stimulating hormone, forty, genetic factor, glands, goiter, gonadal, growth, growth and development, hematocrit, hypothalamus, idiopathic, insomnia, lymphocyte, mental, myxedema, palpitations, pituitary, potassium, puffy, rapid heartbeat, secondary sex, somatotropin (hGH), thick, thyroxine (T4), tissues, tri-iodothyronine (T3), urinary output

Copyright ©2004, Elsevier. All rights reserved.

# ANATOMIC STRUCTURES

*Identify the following structures of the endocrine system.*

1. Major glands of the normal endocrine system

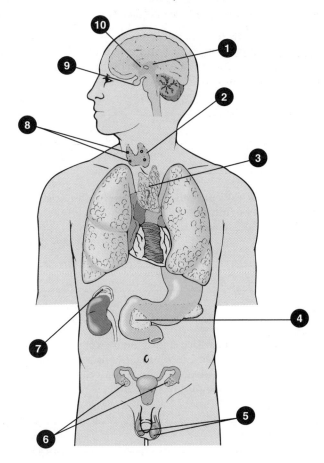

(1) _pineal gland_

(2) _thyroid gland_

(3) _thymus gland_

(4) _pancreas_

(5) _testes (male)_

(6) _ovaries (female)_

(7) _adrenal gland_

(8) _parathyroid glands_

(9) _pituitary gland_

(10) _hypothalamus_

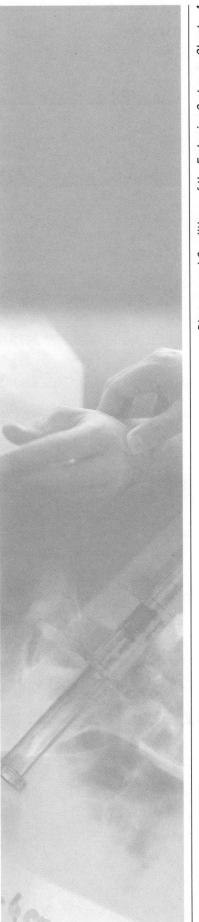

Copyright ©2004, Elsevier. All rights reserved.

# PATIENT SCREENING

*For each scenario below, explain how and why you would schedule an appointment or suggest a referral based on the patient's reported symptoms.* **First, review the "Guidelines for Patient-Screening Exercises" found on page iv in the "Introduction."**

1. A male patient calls for an appointment. He reports experiencing the sudden onset of excessive thirst and urination. He says that he is thirsty all the time and cannot seem to get enough to drink. How do you respond to this phone call?

_____

_____

_____

2. A female patient calls the office and says she thinks she has swelling in her neck and is beginning to experience difficulty swallowing. How do you respond to this phone call?

_____

_____

_____

3. An individual calls the office stating he is experiencing periods of rapid heartbeat and palpitations, insomnia, nervousness, and excitability. He states that despite excessive appetite and food ingestion, he is losing weight. How do you respond to this call?

_____

_____

_____

4. A woman calls the office stating that her husband, who has been diagnosed with diabetes, is experiencing excessive thirst, nausea, drowsiness, and abdominal pain. She just noticed a fruity odor on his breath. She wants to know what to do. How do you respond to this call?

_____

_____

_____

5. A patient calls the office saying she has started experiencing weight loss, excessive thirst, excessive hunger, and frequent urination. She also tells you her mother and Aunt have diabetes. She says she just does not feel right. How do you respond to this call?

_____

_____

_____

Copyright ©2004, Elsevier. All rights reserved.

# PATIENT TEACHING

*For each scenario that follows, outline the appropriate patient teaching you would per-form. First, review the "Guidelines for Patient-Teaching Exercises" found on page iv in the "Introduction."*

1. **ACROMEGALY**
   A diagnosis of acromegaly has been confirmed. The physician (an endocrinologist) has printed materials concerning the disorder. You have been instructed to review the material with the patient and his or her family. How do you handle this patient-teaching opportunity?

   _____

   _____

   _____

2. **DIABETES INSIPIDUS**
   A diagnosis of diabetes insipidus has been confirmed. You are instructed to use available printed material to discuss treatment guidelines with the patient. How do you handle this patient-teaching opportunity?

   _____

   _____

   _____

3. **GRAVES DISEASE**
   An individual with Graves disease has been noncompliant with prescribed medications and has experienced an exacerbation of the condition. The physician has decided the patient requires additional information about the disorder. You are instructed to review the printed materials and guidelines with the patient. How do you handle this patient-teaching opportunity?

   _____

   _____

   _____

4. **HYPOTHYROIDISM**
   A diagnosis of hypothyroidism has just been confirmed. The physician has prescribed a thyroid replacement drug with instructions to take the med-ication as directed and to schedule a checkup in 6 weeks. Additionally, the patient has been told to contact the physician if he or she experiences a rapid heartbeat. How do you handle this patient-teaching opportunity?

   _____

   _____

   _____

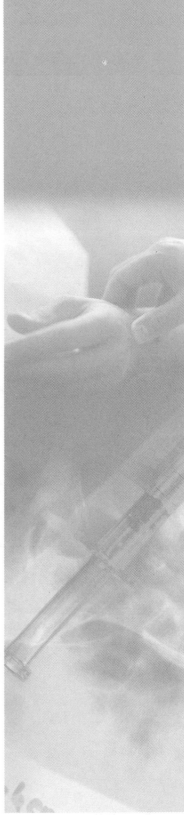

Copyright ©2004, Elsevier. All rights reserved.

5. **DIABETES MELLITUS**

A previously diagnosed individual with diabetes mellitus has been having difficulty maintaining therapeutic glucose levels. You are instructed to provide instructional material concerning the importance of monitoring glucose levels, as well as possible complications of the disorder. How would you handle this patient-teaching opportunity?

_____

_____

_____

## ESSAY QUESTION

*Write a response to the following question or statement. Use a separate sheet of paper if more space is needed.*

Explain the symptoms and treatment for hypoglycemia. Why is this condition considered serious?

_____

_____

_____

_____

_____

_____

_____

_____

_____

_____

_____

_____

_____

_____

_____

_____

_____

_____

Copyright ©2004, Elsevier. All rights reserved.

# CERTIFICATION EXAMINATION REVIEW

*Circle the letter of the choice that best completes the statement or answers the question.*

1. Acromegaly is caused from a hypersecretion of human growth hormone (hGH) that occurs
   a. After puberty
   b. Before puberty
   c. At birth
   d. None of the above

2. Inadequate amounts of dietary iodine may be the cause of
   a. Graves disease
   b. A simple nontoxic goiter
   c. Addison disease
   d. None of the above

3. A calculated diet and exercise, blood and urine testing, and insulin administration are treatments for
   a. Gestational diabetes
   b. Diabetes insipidus
   c. Diabetes mellitus
   d. None of the above

4. Hyperglycemia, thirst, nausea, vomiting, and dry skin are all symptoms of
   a. Diabetic coma
   b. Insulin shock
   c. Gestational diabetes
   c. None of the above

5. Any dysfunction of the endocrine system results in a/an
   a. Increase secretion of hormones
   b. Decrease in secretion of hormones
   c. Both of the above
   d. None of the above

6. A person experiencing insulin shock requires
   a. Insulin
   b. Glucose
   c. Simple sugar
   d. None of the above

7. Severe hypothyroidism or myxedema has its onset during
   a. Infancy
   b. Older childhood
   c. Adulthood
   d. Both b and c

8. Dwarfism is the abnormal underdevelopment of the body or hypopituitarism that occurs in
   a. Infancy
   b. Older childhood
   c. Adulthood
   d. None of the above

9. Gigantism is caused from a hypersecretion of human growth hormone that occurs
   a. Before puberty
   b. After puberty
   c. At any age
   d. At birth

Copyright ©2004, Elsevier. All rights reserved.

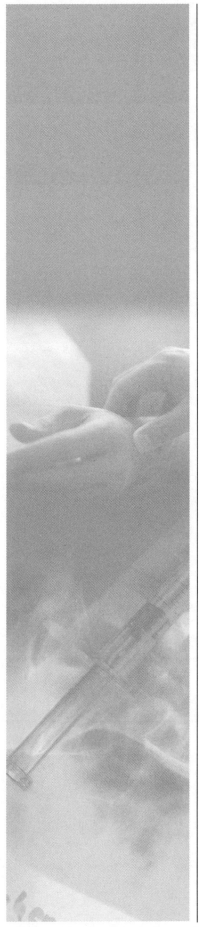

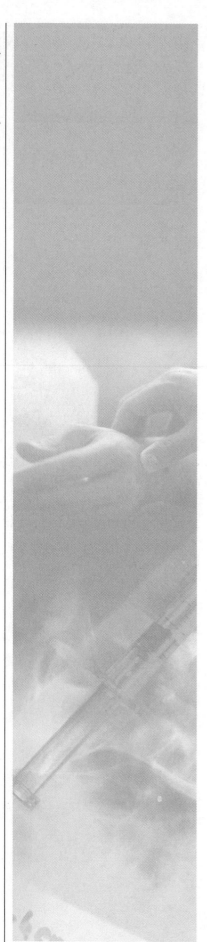

10. Cushing syndrome causes symptoms of
    a. Weight loss, rash, and alopecia
    b. Fatigue, muscle weakness, and changes in body appearance
    c. A bright red rash and itching
    d. None of the above

11. Evaluation for cancer of the thyroid gland should be sought if the patient has
    a. A painless lump or nodule on the thyroid gland
    b. A painful lump or nodule on the thyroid gland
    c. Either a or b
    d. None of the above

12. Addison disease has a gradual onset and involves the
    a. Parathyroid glands
    b. Pancreas
    c. Adrenal glands
    d. Thyroid gland

Copyright ©2004, Elsevier. All rights reserved.

# CHAPTER 5

# Diseases and Disorders of the Eye and Ear

## WORD DEFINITIONS

*Define the following basic medical terms:*

1. Arteritis

2. Bilateral — Relating to the left + right

3. Dilated — to enlarge

4. Edema — abnormal/excessive amount of serous fluid in connective tissue

5. Excision — Surgical removal

6. Hemorrhage — a copious discharge of blood from the blood vessels

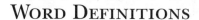
7. Hyperopia — can see things far but not near

8. Hypertrophied — to enlarge in size

9. Intracranial — situated in the cranium

10. Intraocular — implanted in the eyeball

11. Meningitis — inflamation of the meninges

12. Myopia — nearsightedness — can see things close but not far

13. Postoperative — following an operation

14. Proliferative — growing by rapid production of new parts cells buds or offspring

15. Strabismus — inability of 7 eye to attain binocular vision w/one other y/c of impalance of the muscles of the eyeball — cross eyed

16. Systemic — Relating to a system

17. Topical — designed for or involving local application to or surface action on a bodily part

18. Vertigo — disordered state which is associated w/various disorders; seem to whirl dizzily

Copyright ©2004, Elsevier. All rights reserved.

# GLOSSARY TERMS

*Define the following chapter glossary terms:*

1. Amblyopia — reduced vision in an eye w/o a detectable organic lesion

2. Analgesics — relief of pain

3. Ankylosis — immobility of a joint

4. Audiogram — record of a hearing test

5. Diplopia — double vision

6. Histoplasmosis — systemic respiratory disease caused by a fungus

7. Laser photocoagulation — coagulation of the blood vessels in the eye using a laser

8. Macula — small spot or a colored area

9. Photophobia — unusual sensitivity to light

10. Purulent — containing pus

11. Seborrhea — excessive secretion of sebum from sebaceous glands

12. Tinnitus — ringing in the ears

13. Tonometry — measurement of intraocular pressure

14. Toxoplasmosis — disease caused by infection w/ protozoa found in many mamals

15. Tympanic membrane — eardrum

# SHORT ANSWER

*Answer the following questions:*

1. Identify the concentric layers of the eyeball that are its primary structure.

2. Name the colorless transparent structure located on the front of the eye.

3. List the way that hearing loss is classified.

4. Explain the symptoms associated with otosclerosis.

5. Name the canal that leads from the middle ear to the nasopharynx.

Copyright ©2004, Elsevier. All rights reserved.

6. Identify the structure in the ear that is responsible for helping a person maintain balance.

_____

7. Cite the shape of the normal eyeball.

_____

8. Name the sensory receptive cells in the retina that make the detection of color and fine detail possible.

_____

9. Identify the waxlike secretion that is produced by the glands of the external ear canal.

_____

10. Name the jellylike fluid found in the cavity behind the lens of the eye.

_____

11. Name the internal elastic structure of the eye that focuses images both near and far.

_____

12. What is the cause of a cholesteatoma?

_____

13. If the eyeball is abnormally short, name the condition that occurs.

_____

14. If the eyeball is abnormally long, name the condition that occurs.

_____

15. Identify the cause of astigmatism.

_____

16. List the primary symptoms of refractive errors.

_____

17. Name the most common type of nystagmus.

_____

18. Identify the bacteria that are the common cause of styes.

_____

19. List the symptoms of keratitis.

_____

20. Explain the most common cause of cataracts.

_____

Copyright ©2004, Elsevier. All rights reserved.

21. Is there a cure for macular degeneration?

_____

22. Identify the disorder of the retinal blood vessels that may develop in a person who has diabetes.

_____

23. Explain the steps that may be used to remove impacted cerumen.

_____

_____

24. List the four most common causes of a ruptured eardrum.

_____

_____

## FILL IN THE BLANKS

*Fill in the blanks with the correct terms. A Word List has been provided. Words used twice are indicated with a (2).*

1. The iris or colored portion of the eye helps regulate the amount of

_____ that enters the eye.

2. The large cavity behind the lens of the eye contains a jellylike fluid called

the _____ _____.

3. Four main refractive errors that result when the eye is unable to focus

light effectively on the retina are _____,

_____, _____, and

_____.

4. The patient with myopia can see objects that are near but experiences

difficulty seeing objects that are _distant_.

5. _Strabismus_ is the failure of the eyes to look in the same

direction at the same time, which primarily occurs because of

_weakness_ in the nerves stimulating the muscles that con-

trol the _position_ of the eye.

6. In _esotropia_, both eyes turn inward; in exotropia, both

eyes turn outward.

50

Copyright ©2004, Elsevier. All rights reserved.

7. The symptoms of a stye are _pain_, _swelling_, _redness_, and formation of pus at the site.

8. Keratitis is frequently caused by an infection resulting from the _herpes simplex_ virus.

9. Allergies or exposure to _smoke_, dust, or _chemicals_ can cause nonulcerative blepharitis.

10. Blepharoptosis occurs at any _age_, is often _familial_, and if severe, blocks the _vision_ of the affected eye.

11. Infection, either _____ or _____, can cause conjunctivitis.

12. A corneal abrasion or ulceration is the painful loss of _surface_ epithelium, or outer layers of the _cornea_.

13. A cataract may become visible, giving the pupil a _white_, opaque appearance.

14. The best way to detect glaucoma is to have periodic _____ _____ examinations.

15. Common symptoms of ear diseases and conditions that should receive medical attention include _hearing loss_, ear _pain_ or _pressure tinnitus_ vertigo, nausea, and _vomiting_.

16. Impacted _cerumen_ may harden and block sound waves resulting in decreased hearing.

17. Otitis _media_ is the most frequent reason for visits to the physician by children.

## WORD LIST

age, astigmatism, bacterial, cerumen, chemicals, cornea, distant, esotropia, familial, hearing loss, herpes simplex, hyperopia, light, media, myopia, pain (2), position, presbyopia, pressure, routine ophthalmic, redness, smoke, strabismus, surface, swelling, tinnitus, viral, vision, vitreous humor, vomiting, weakness, white

Copyright ©2004, Elsevier. All rights reserved.

# ANATOMIC STRUCTURES

*Identify the structures in the following anatomic diagrams.*

1. Normal eye

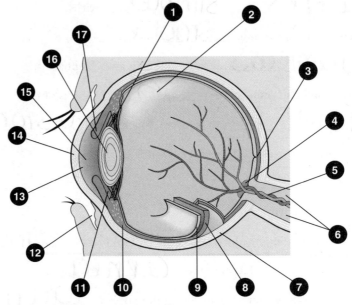

(1)   Suspensory ligaments

(2)   Vitreous body & humor

(3)   fovea centralis

(4)   Optic disk

(5)   retinal artery & vein

(6)   Optic nerve

(7)   Sclera

(8)   Choroid

(9)   retina

(10)   ciliary body

(11)   posterior chamber

(12)   conjunctival sac

(13)   anterior cavity filled w/ aqueous humor

(14)   cornea

(15)   pupil

(16)   lens

(17)   iris

Copyright ©2004, Elsevier. All rights reserved.

2. The visual pathway

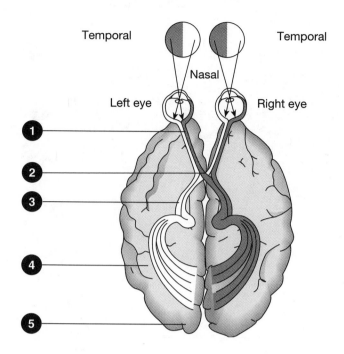

Left visual field   Right visual field

Temporal               Temporal

Nasal

Left eye         Right eye

(1)   Optic nerve

(2)   Optic chiasm

(3)   Optic tract

(4)   brain

(5)   Occipital lobe

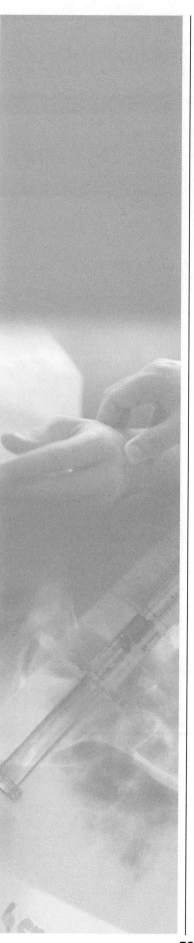

Copyright ©2004, Elsevier. All rights reserved.

3. Normal ear

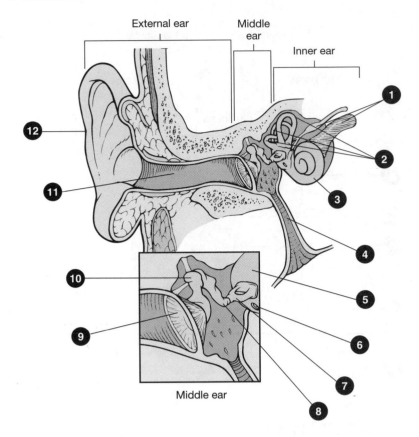

Middle ear

(1) Vestibulocochlear nerve
(2) Semicircular canals
(3) Cochlea
(4) Eustachian
(5) Oval window
(6) Round window
(7) Stapes
(8) Incus
(9) Tympanic membrane
(10) Malleus
(11) External auditory canal
(12) Pinna (auricle)

Copyright ©2004, Elsevier. All rights reserved.

4. Labyrinth or inner ear

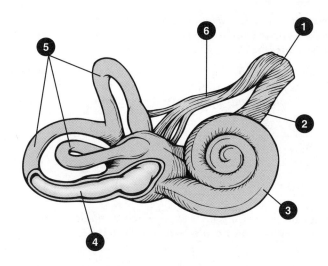

(1) _Vestibulocochlear nerve_
(2) _Cochlear nerve_
(3) _Cochlea_
(4) _endolymph_
(5) _Semicircular canals_
(6) _Vestibular nerve_

Copyright ©2004, Elsevier. All rights reserved.

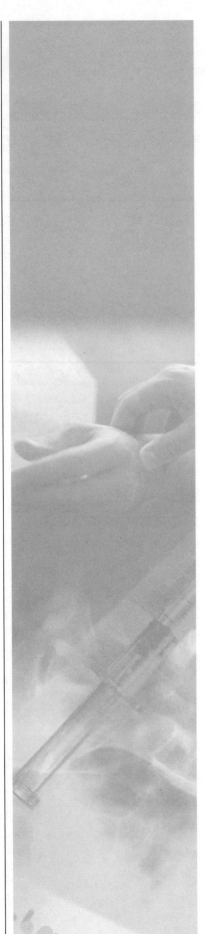

# PATIENT SCREENING

*For each scenario that follows, explain how and why you would schedule an appointment or suggest a referral based on the patient's reported symptoms.* ***First, review the "Guidelines for Patient-Screening Exercises" found on page iv in the "Introduction."***

1. A patient calls in describing a sensation of constantly having something in her right eye. She also states the pain and tearing prevent her from wearing her contact lens in that eye. How do you handle this call?

   _____

   _____

   _____

2. A patient calls in advising he is experiencing changes in his vision and a sensitivity to light. How do you handle this call?

   _____

   _____

   _____

   _____

3. A patient calls in reporting she is experiencing reduced vision, especially loss of sharpness in her central vision. How do you respond to this call?

   _____

   _____

   _____

   _____

4. A patient calls the office and tells you he suddenly is having flashes of light along with floating spots in the left eye. How do you respond to this call?

   _____

   _____

   _____

   _____

5. A father calls the office reporting his child is experiencing ear pain, has a fever, and appears to have diminished hearing. How do you handle this call?

   _____

   _____

   _____

   _____

Copyright ©2004, Elsevier. All rights reserved.

# PATIENT TEACHING

*For each scenario below, outline the appropriate patient teaching you would perform.*
***First, review the "Guidelines for Patient-Teaching Exercises" found on page iv in the***
***"Introduction."***

1. STYE

   A patient has just been diagnosed with having a stye on the eyelid. Eye
   compresses and topical antibiotics have been prescribed. You are
   instructed to provide the patient with instructions regarding the application of compresses and topical eye medications. How would you handle
   this patient-teaching opportunity?

   _____

   _____

   _____

   _____

2. KERATITIS

   A diagnosis of keratitis has been made. The physician instructs you to use
   printed materials to explain proper administration of eye medications
   and to reinforce the importance of good handwashing before touching
   an eye. How do you handle this patient-teaching opportunity?

   _____

   _____

   _____

   _____

3. CONJUNCTIVITIS

   A patient with conjunctivitis has been advised to use cool compresses on
   both eyes for comfort. Topical ophthalmic medications have also been
   prescribed for therapeutic treatment. You have been instructed to advise
   the patient on how to apply the cool compresses and medications. How
   would you handle this patient-teaching opportunity?

   _____

   _____

   _____

   _____

4. GLAUCOMA

   A patient has just been diagnosed with glaucoma. (Type is insignificant in
   this situation.) You have been instructed to discuss treatment regimen
   with the patient. How do you handle this patient-teaching opportunity?

   _____

   _____

   _____

   _____

Copyright ©2004, Elsevier. All rights reserved.

5. **IMPACTED CERUMEN**

A child has been experiencing diminished hearing and has been complaining of slight pain in the ears. A diagnosis of impacted cerumen is made. You are instructed to reinforce appropriate cleansing of the ear canal. How do you handle this patient-teaching opportunity?

_____

_____

_____

_____

# ESSAY QUESTION

*Write a response to the following question or statement. Use a separate sheet of paper if more space is needed.*

Discuss the symptoms, causes, and treatment for a ruptured tympanic membrane.

_____

_____

_____

_____

_____

_____

_____

_____

_____

_____

_____

_____

_____

_____

_____

_____

_____

Copyright ©2004, Elsevier. All rights reserved.

# CERTIFICATION EXAMINATION REVIEW

*Circle the letter of the choice that best completes the statement or answers the question.*

1. When the eye is unable to focus light effectively, which of the following may result?
   a. Hyperopia
   b. Myopia
   c. Presbyopia
   d. All of the above

2. Laser surgery, contact lenses, and eyeglasses would be treatment for
   a. Folliculitis
   b. Conjunctivitis
   c. Refractive errors
   d. All of the above

3. A stye is an:
   a. Inflammation of the conjunctiva
   b. Inflammation of the hair follicle of the eyelid
   c. Inflammation of the retina
   d. None of the above

4. Conjunctivitis is an
   a. Inflammation of the thin membrane covering the visible portion of the sclera and lining the inside of the eyelids
   b. Inflammation of the hair follicle of the eyelid
   c. Inflammation of the retina
   d. None of the above

5. Infection, irritation, allergies, or chemicals may be the cause of
   a. Hyperopia
   b. Myopia
   c. Conjunctivitis
   d. All of the above

6. Glaucoma is a major cause of _____ in the United States.
   a. Blindness
   b. Hearing loss
   c. Retinal detachment
   d. None of the above

7. Otosclerosis is an ankylosing of the
   a. Labyrinth
   b. Stapes
   c. Eyelid
   d. None of the above

8. Labyrinthitis is an inflammation of the
   a. Stapes
   b. Conjunctiva
   c. Semicircular canal
   d. None of the above

9. Otosclerosis, impacted cerumen, and otitis media may be the cause of
   a. Conductive hearing loss
   b. Sensorineural hearing loss
   c. Both a and b
   d. Neither a or b

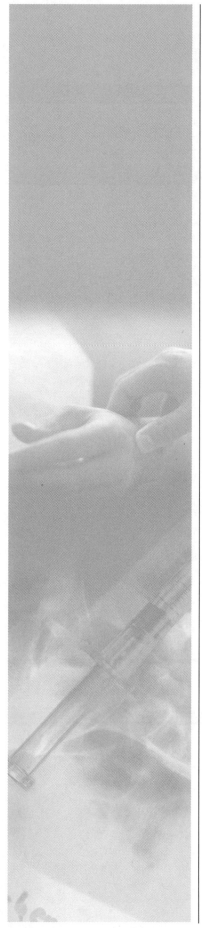

Copyright ©2004, Elsevier. All rights reserved.

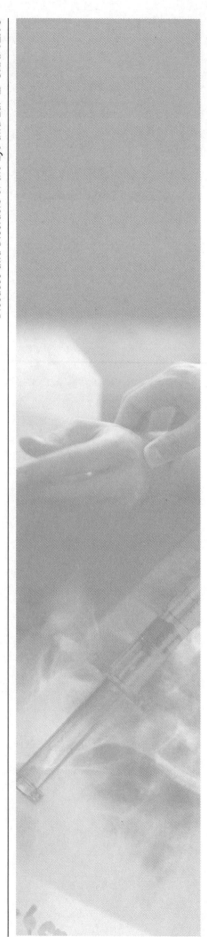

10. The internal _____ of the eye is elastic and can focus images both near and far.
    a. Sclera
    b. Iris
    c. Lens
    d. None of the above

Copyright ©2004, Elsevier. All rights reserved.

# CHAPTER 6

# Diseases and Conditions of the Integumentary System

## WORD DEFINITIONS

*Define the following basic medical terms:*

1. Anemia — condition in which the blood is deficient in Red blood cells

2. Colic

3. Edema — excessive amount of serious fluid in the connective tissue

4. Epidemic

5. Erythema — abnormal redness of skin due to capillary congestion (inflamation)

6. Excision — surgical removal

7. Hyperplastic — abnormal increase in the elements composing a part

8. Hypertrophic — relating to or affected with hypertrophy

9. Lesion — abnormal change in structure of a organ due to injury / disease

10. Peripheral — located near a periphery or surface part

11. Psychosis — serious mental disorder

12. Sebaceous — secreting sebum

13. Spore

14. Superficial — located near the surface

15. Unilateral — affecting 1 side of the body

Copyright ©2004, Elsevier. All rights reserved.

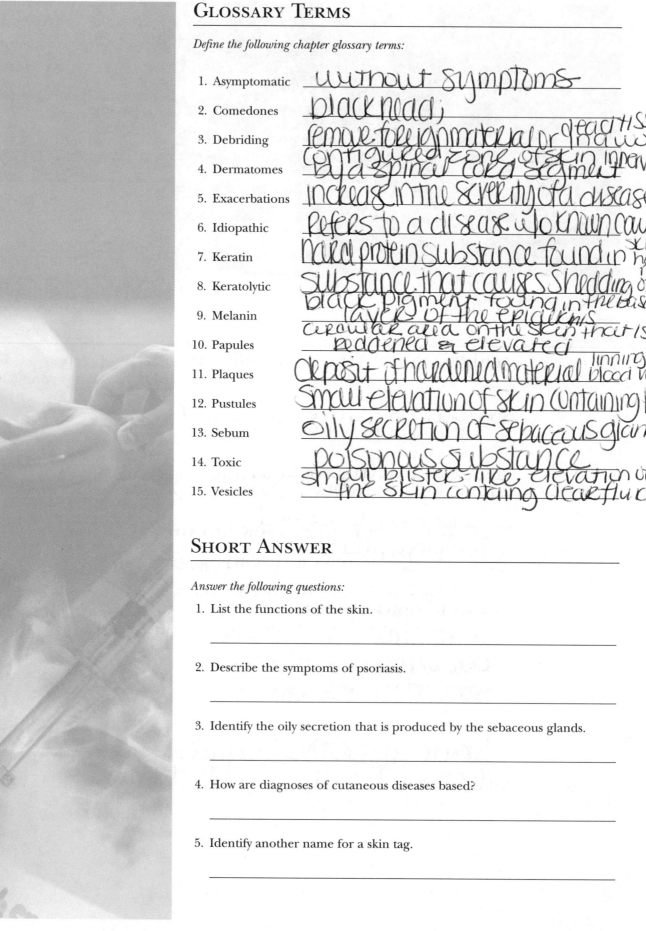

# GLOSSARY TERMS

*Define the following chapter glossary terms:*

1. Asymptomatic — without symptoms

2. Comedones — blackhead;

3. Debriding — remove foreign material or dead tissue of a wound

4. Dermatomes — configured zone of skin innervated by a spinal cord segment

5. Exacerbations — increase in the severity of a disease

6. Idiopathic — refers to a disease w/o known cause

7. Keratin — hard protein substance found in skin, hair, nails.

8. Keratolytic — substance that causes shedding of skin

9. Melanin — black pigment found in the basal layer of the epidermis

10. Papules — circular area on the skin that is reddened & elevated

11. Plaques — deposit of hardened material linning the blood vessel

12. Pustules — small elevation of skin containing pus

13. Sebum — oily secretion of sebaceous glands

14. Toxic — poisonous substance

15. Vesicles — small blister-like elevation of the skin containing clear fluid

# SHORT ANSWER

*Answer the following questions:*

1. List the functions of the skin.

2. Describe the symptoms of psoriasis.

3. Identify the oily secretion that is produced by the sebaceous glands.

4. How are diagnoses of cutaneous diseases based?

5. Identify another name for a skin tag.

Copyright ©2004, Elsevier. All rights reserved.

6. Which type of skin cancer is the most prevalent form of cancer worldwide?

_____

7. Identify the bacteria that cause impetigo.

_____

8. List examples of dermatophytosis.

_____

9. List examples of common benign skin tumors.

_____

10. Identify the other name for a mole.

_____

11. Are keloids benign or malignant?

_____

12. When do keloids form?

_____

13. At what age will cradle cap resolve if left untreated?

_____

14. Name the test that is used to identify specific irritants or allergens that cause contact dermatitis.

_____

15. List three things that may cause eczema to flare up.

_____

16. Explain the goal of treatment for psoriasis.

_____

17. Identify the other name for herpes zoster.

_____

18. Cite the other name for a furuncle.

_____

19. Which area of the body is usually affected by cellulitis?

_____

20. Describe the appearance of a ringworm lesion.

_____

Copyright ©2004, Elsevier. All rights reserved.

21. Identify the area of the body affected by tinea unguium.

_____

22. Identify the area of the body affected by tinea pedis.

_____

23. Which sex is at more at risk for tinea cruris?

_____

24. Cite the statistics for lesion occurrence of basal cell carcinoma on the face.

_____

25. Cite the statistics for 5-year survival rate of nonmelanoma skin cancer.

_____

26. Name the special cells in the skin that produce melanin.

_____

27. What color eyes would a person with albinism have?

_____

28. Will alopecia resulting from the aging process or heredity improve?

_____

# FILL IN THE BLANKS

*Fill in the blanks with the correct terms. A Word List has been provided.*

1. The skin is one of the ___largest___ organs in size.
2. The dermis is the ___middle___ layer of the skin.
3. The ___epidermis___ is the outer thin layer of the skin that is responsible for the production of ___keratin___ and ___melanin___.
4. The third layer of the skin is the ___subcutaneous layer___, a thick, fat-containing section that provides ___insulation___ for the body against heat loss.
5. Seborrheic dermatitis can be treated effectively with topical ___hydrocortisone___ cream.

Copyright ©2004, Elsevier. All rights reserved.

6. Urticaria, or ___hives___, is associated with symptoms of severe ___itching___, followed by the appearance of ___redness___ and an area of swelling.

7. Albinism is a rare ___inherited___ condition.

8. Melasma occurs in some women during ___hormonal___ changes. The condition disappears after ___pregnancy___ or when oral contraceptive use is ___discontinued___.

9. Hemangiomas are ___benign___ lesions of proliferating ___blood___ ___vessels___ that produce a ___red___, blue, or ___purple___ color.

10. Seborrheic ___warts___ are not true warts but are ___round___ or oval patches of ___(darkly)___ pigmented skin.

11. A fungal infection that causes patches of flaky light or dark skin to develop on the trunk of the body is called ___pityriasis___.

12. The treatment that is showing promise for male pattern baldness is ___minoxidil (Rogaine)___ preparations used topically in cream and spray forms.

**WORD LIST**

benign, blood vessels, discontinued, epidermis, hives, hormonal, hydrocortisone, inherited, insulation, itching, keratin, largest, melanin, middle, minoxidil (Rogaine), pityriasis, pregnancy, purple, red, redness, round, subcutaneous layer, warts

Copyright ©2004, Elsevier. All rights reserved.

# ANATOMIC STRUCTURES

*Identify the structures of the following anatomic diagram.*

1. Normal skin

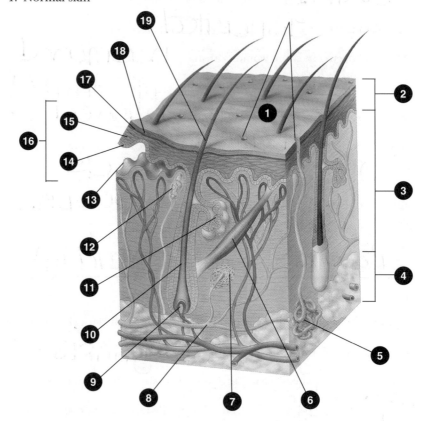

(1) opening of sweat glands

(2) epidermis

(3) dermis

(4) subcutaneous layer

(5) sweat gland

(6) arrector pili muscle

(7) pacinian corpuscle

(8) cutaneous nerve

(9) papilla of hair

(10) hair follicle

(11) subaceous gland

(12) meissner corpuscle

(13) dermal papilla

(14) stratum basale

(15) stratum spinosum

(16) stratum germinativum

(17) stratum granulosum

(18) stratum corneum

(19) hair shaft

Copyright ©2004, Elsevier. All rights reserved.

# PATIENT SCREENING

*For each scenario below, explain how and why you would schedule an appointment or suggest a referral based on the patient's reported symptoms.* **First, review the "Guidelines for Patient-Screening Exercises" found on page iv in the "Introduction."**

1. The mother of a 10-year-old child calls in to request an appointment for her daughter who has seeping eruptions on her elbows and knees. She also says the child is experiencing constant itching. How do you handle this phone call?

_____

_____

_____

2. A patient calls complaining of severe itching of the arms, hands, and trunk that is accompanied by a red rash. This situation has occurred in the past 2 hours and is getting progressively worse. How do you handle this call?

_____

_____

_____

3. A patient's wife calls in stating her husband has the onset of excruciating pain on the right side in the middle of the trunk. She says it appears there are small blisterlike eruptions over the area on the right side of the body. She says he needs help as soon as possible. How do you handle this call?

_____

_____

_____

4. A mother calls reporting her daughter has just come home from school with areas on her legs and arms having small blisters that are surrounded with small blisterlike formations. She says the child is continuously scratching the areas, and they are getting worse. She requests an appointment for the next morning, saying she will keep the child home from school until seen by the physician. When do you schedule the child to be seen?

_____

_____

_____

5. A female patient calls stating she has a sore on her right shoulder that has refused to heal completely and has occurrences of bleeding. She states that the sore is about an inch in diameter and has irregular edges. She requests an appointment for assessment of the sore. How do you schedule the appointment?

_____

_____

_____

Copyright ©2004, Elsevier. All rights reserved.

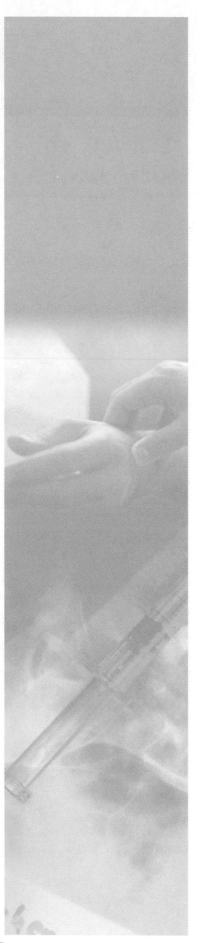

# PATIENT TEACHING

*For each scenario below, outline the appropriate patient teaching you would perform.*
***First, review the "Guidelines for Patient-Teaching Exercises" found on page iv in the***
***"Introduction."***

1. **CONTACT DERMATITIS**

   A patient has just been seen for the second time in 3 weeks for contact dermatitis. The area is now showing signs of a developing infection. The physician instructs you to reinforce his instructions about avoiding the trigger substance, as well as trying to avoid scratching the area. How do you handle the patient-teaching opportunity?

   _____

   _____

   _____

2. **ACNE**

   A teenage patient has experienced an exacerbation of acne. Topical and oral medications have been prescribed. You have been instructed to provide the patient with printed information regarding the treatment of acne. How do you handle this patient-teaching opportunity?

   _____

   _____

   _____

3. **DERMATOPHYTOSIS**

   A patient has been diagnosed with athlete's foot. You have been instructed to provide him or her with printed information regarding the treatment of this condition. How do you handle this patient-teaching opportunity?

   _____

   _____

   _____

4. **SCABIES AND PEDICULOSIS**

   A patient was sent home from school with the possibility of head lice. You have been instructed to provide the parents and patient with printed information regarding this condition. How will you handle this patient-teaching opportunity?

   _____

   _____

   _____

Copyright ©2004, Elsevier. All rights reserved.

5. **SKIN CANCER**

A patient has been seen for several skin lesions. Some are diagnosed as being benign. One is suspicious in nature, and the patient is referred to a dermatologist for further assessment and treatment. You are instructed to provide the patient with printed information concerning skin lesions and to encourage the use of sunscreen. How do you handle this patient-teaching opportunity?

_____

_____

_____

# ESSAY QUESTION

*Write a response to the following question or statement. Use a separate sheet of paper if more space is needed.*

Describe the cause, symptoms, and treatment for herpes zoster (shingles).

_____

_____

_____

_____

_____

_____

_____

_____

_____

_____

_____

_____

# CERTIFICATION EXAMINATION REVIEW

*Circle the letter of the choice that best completes the statement or answers the question.*

1. *Streptococcus* or *Staphylococcus* are bacteria that can cause the skin infection called
   a. Psoriasis
   b. Eczema
   c. Impetigo
   d. None of the above

Copyright ©2004, Elsevier. All rights reserved.

2. Atopic dermatitis is another name for _____. This is a skin infection that tends to occur in people who have a family history of allergic conditions.
   a. Psoriasis
   b. Eczema
   c. Impetigo
   d. None of the above

3. Cradle cap is a type of seborrheic dermatitis that is seen in
   a. Infants
   b. Teenagers
   c. Adults
   d. All of the above

4. Good skin care, early ambulation, and position changes every 2 hours are all considered preventative measures to reduce the likelihood of developing _____ _____
   a. Herpes zoster
   b. Decubitus ulcers
   c. Atopic dermatitis
   d. None of the above

5. The two most common parasitic infections to infest humans are
   a. Herpes zoster
   b. Atopic dermatitis
   c. Scabies and pediculosis
   d. None of the above

6. Malignant melanoma is the most serious type of
   a. Skin cancer
   b. Fungal infection
   c. Parasitic infection
   d. None of the above

7. A furuncle is an abscess that involves the entire hair follicle and
   a. Underlying muscle tissue
   b. The epidermis
   c. The adjacent subcutaneous tissue
   d. None of the above

8. Manifestations of dermatophytosis include
   a. Tinea capitis, tinea corporis, tinea pedis, and tinea cruris
   b. Scabies and pediculosis
   c. Albinism and vitiligo
   d. All of the above

9. The patient with psoriasis will exhibit symptoms of
   a. A fine red rash that itches
   b. Large furuncles and a fine red rash
   c. Thick, flaky red patches of various sizes, covered with white silvery scales
   d. None of the above

10. The transmission of lice and scabies from one person to another is
   a. Difficult
   b. Easy with close physical contact
   c. Only possible if two people live in the same house
   d. None of the above

Copyright ©2004, Elsevier. All rights reserved.

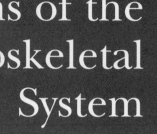

# CHAPTER 7

# Diseases and Conditions of the Musculoskeletal System

## WORD DEFINITIONS

*Define the following basic medical terms:*

1. Adjacent

2. Bacterium

3. Bunionectomy   *Surgical excission of a bunion*

4. Calcanean   *relating to the heal*

5. Calcification

6. Collagen

7. Edematous   *affected w/ edema*

8. Extension   *stretching of a dislocated limb to bring it back to its place*

9. Fasciitis   *inflamation of a fascia*

10. Flexion

11. Hyperbaric oxygen treatment

12. Hyperostosis   *excessive growth of bone tissue*

13. Intraarticular   *occuring within a joint*

14. Laxity   *state of being loose*

15. Osteotomy   *piece of bone excised*

16. Plantar   *relating to the sole of the foot*

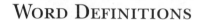

Copyright ©2004, Elsevier. All rights reserved.

## GLOSSARY TERMS

*Define the following chapter glossary terms:*

1. Abscess — localized collection of pus surrounded by swollen tissue

2. Arthrodesis — immobilization of a joint accomplished surgically

3. Arthroplasty — surgical reconstruction or replacement of a diseased joint

4. Cheilectomy — surgical removal of abnormal bone around a joint

5. Closed reduction — non-surgical manipulative reduction of a dislocation/fracture

6. Echocardiographic — ultrasonographic study of the motion of the walls/structures of the ♡

7. Hallux — great toe

8. Hyperuricemia — excessive uric acid levels in the blood

9. Magnetic resonance imaging (MRI) —

10. Metatarsophalangeal — pertaining to the phalanges of the toes metatarsus

11. Open reduction — exposure of a fractured/dislocated bone through a surgical incision to region the bone

12. Osteophytes — bony outgrowth; usually branch shaped

13. Periosteum — fibrous covering of long bones

14. Purulent — containing pus

15. Sclerosing — hardening of a body part

16. Sequestrum — segment of dead bone

17. Skeletal traction —

18. Subluxation — partial dislocation

19. Synovial — pertaining to fluid around a joint

20. Tendinitis — inflammation of a tendon

## SHORT ANSWER

*Answer the following questions:*

1. Identify when shin splints are likely to occur.

2. Cite the cause of fibromyalgia.

Copyright ©2004, Elsevier. All rights reserved.

3. Is there a specific laboratory test to identify whether a patient has fibromyalgia?

_____

4. Name the most common form of arthritis.

_____

5. Describe the rash that sometimes accompanies Lyme disease.

_____

6. Identify the cause of gouty arthritis.

_____

7. Name the hereditary syndrome that affects the connective tissue and causes an abnormal growth of the extremities.

_____

8. Cite the other name for Paget disease.

_____

9. Identify the most common sites of the body affected by Paget disease.

_____

10. Name the most common type of primary bone neoplasm.

_____

11. A deficiency in vitamin D may cause what abnormal metabolic bone disease?

_____

12. Which sex is more likely to be affected by osteoporosis?

_____

13. Name the term for a benign growth filled with a jellylike substance that commonly develops on the back of the wrist and may be caused by repetitive injury.

_____

14. Cite the other name for a hallux valgus.

_____

15. Name the injury that involves the semilunar cartilages in the knee.

_____

16. List the three abnormal curvatures of the spine.

_____

Copyright ©2004, Elsevier. All rights reserved.

17. Identify the structures in the skeletal system affected by osteoarthritis.

_____

_____

18. What year was Lyme disease first detected?

_____

19. List the classic symptoms of bursitis.

_____

_____

20. Name the medication that may be injected into the joint to treat bursitis.

_____

21. Identify the area of the foot that is usually affected by gout.

_____

22. Is Ewing's sarcoma encapsulated?

_____

23. Cite the statistics for overall 5-year survival rate for patients with primary bone cancer.

_____

24. List the terms used to classify sprains.

_____

25. Name the procedure that is used to remove a limb when a peripheral vascular disease has occurred as a result of atherosclerosis and consequent gangrene, trauma, malignancy, or congenital defects.

_____

26. Are muscle tumors frequently diagnosed?

_____

27. Which area of the body is affected when a person has plantar fasciitis?

_____

28. What can a person do to prevent heel spurs?

_____

_____

Copyright ©2004, Elsevier. All rights reserved.

# FILL IN THE BLANKS

*Fill in the blanks with the correct terms. A Word List has been provided. Words used twice are indicated with a (2).*

1. All movement, including the movement of the ___body___ themselves and of the ___organs___ is performed by ___muscle___ tissue.

2. The three types of muscle tissue are ___muscles___ or skeletal, ___nonstriated___ or smooth, and ___cardiac___.

3. Bones develop through a process called ___osteogenesis___

4. The complete skeleton is formed by the end of the ___third___ month of ___gestation___.

5. Joints are classified according to their ___movement___.

6. ___cartilage___ is a semi-smooth, dense, supporting connective ___tissue___ that is found at the ___ends___ of ___bones___.

7. A patient with fibromyalgia has a relatively low level of the brain nerve chemical ___serotonin___.

8. Bursae are found between _____ and _____ and cover _____ prominences, _____ movement.

9. The most commonly involved bones in osteomyelitic infections are the upper ends of the _____ and _____, the lower end of the _____, and occasionally the _____.

10. Phantom _____ sensation is an unpleasant complication that sometimes follows a(an) _____.

11. Permanent _____ _____ can result from tendon damage.

12. A _____ most commonly develops on the _____ of the wrist as a single, _____ lump, just under the ___surface___ of the skin.

## WORD LIST

amputation, back, body, bones, bony, cardiac, cartilage, ends, facilitating, femur, ganglion, gestation, humerus, limb, movement, muscle atrophy, muscles (2), nonstriated, organs, osteogenesis, serotonin, smooth, striated, surface, tendons, third, tibia, tissue, vertebrae

Copyright ©2004, Elsevier. All rights reserved.

# ANATOMIC STRUCTURES

*Identify the structures of the following anatomic diagrams.*

1. Normal muscular system—anterior view

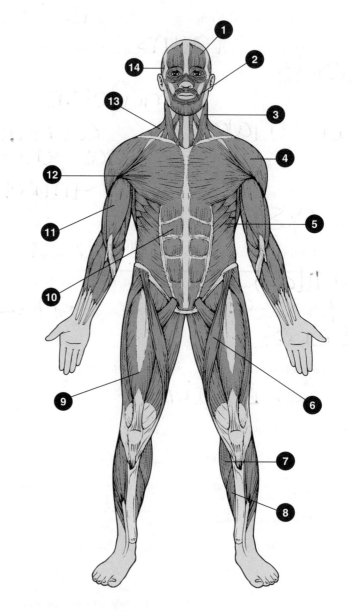

(1) _frontalis_

(2) _masseter_

(3) _sternocleidomastoid_

(4) _Deltoid_

(5) _external oblique_

(6) _Sartorius_

(7) _gastrocnemius_

(8) _Soleus_

(9) _RECTUS FEMORIS_

(10) _RECTUS Abdominis_

(11) _Biceps Brachii_

(12) _Pectoralis major_

(13) _trapezius_

(14) _temporalis_

Copyright ©2004, Elsevier. All rights reserved.

2. Normal muscular system—posterior view

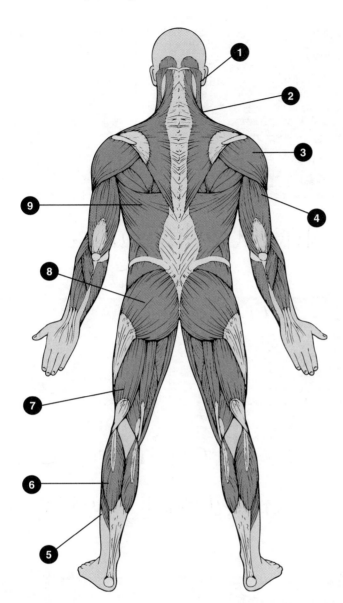

(1) sternocleidomastoid
(2) trapezius
(3) Deltoid
(4) triceps bracnii
(5) soleus
(6) gastrocnemius
(7) Biceps femoris
(8) gluteus maximus
(9) Latissimus dorsi

Copyright ©2004, Elsevier. All rights reserved.

3. Types of muscles

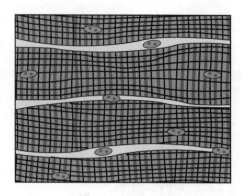 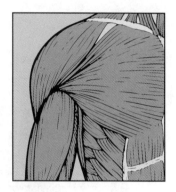

striated (skeletal) muscle

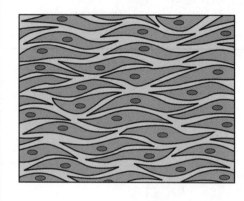 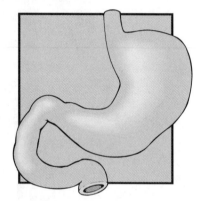

nonstriated (smooth) muscle

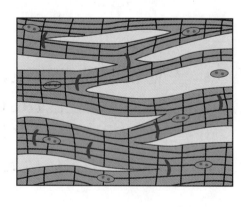 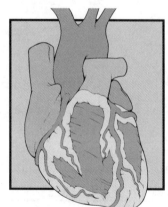

Cardiac muscle

Copyright ©2004, Elsevier. All rights reserved.

4. Normal skeletal system—anterior view

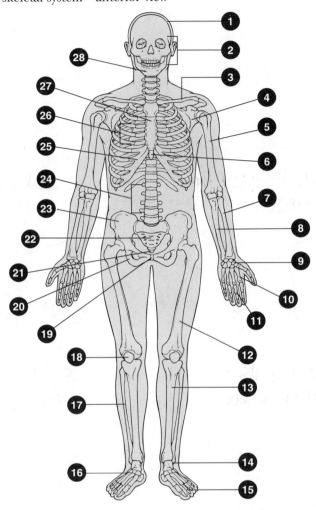

(1) Cranium
(2) facial bones
(3) clavicle
(4) scapula
(5) Humerus
(6) Xiphoid process
(7) Radius
(8) Ulna
(9) carpals
(10) metacarpals
(11) phalanges
(12) femur
(13) patella
(14) tarsals
(15) met phalanges
(16) metatarsals
(17) tibia
(18) patella
(19) pubis
(20) Ischium
(21) coccyx
(22) Sacrum
(23) Ilium
(24) vertebral column
(25) costal cartilage
(26) Ribs
(27) sternum
(28) mad

Copyright ©2004, Elsevier. All rights reserved.

5. Examples of types of joints

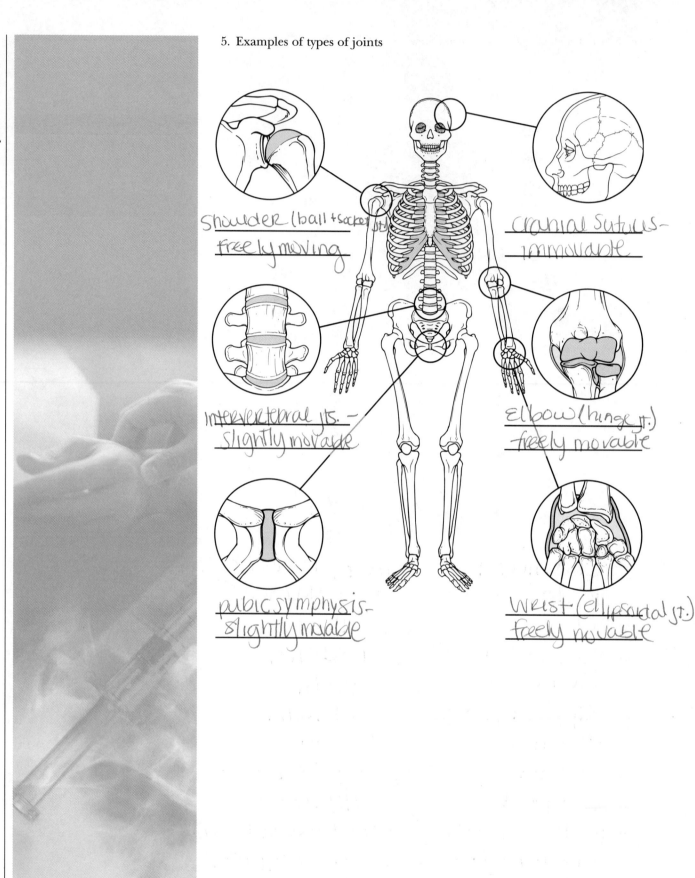

Shoulder (ball + socket jt)
freely moving

cranial sutures-
immovable

intervertebral jts. -
slightly movable

Elbow (hinge jt.)
freely movable

pubic symphysis-
slightly movable

wrist (ellipsoidal jt.)
freely movable

Copyright ©2004, Elsevier. All rights reserved.

6. Types of fractures

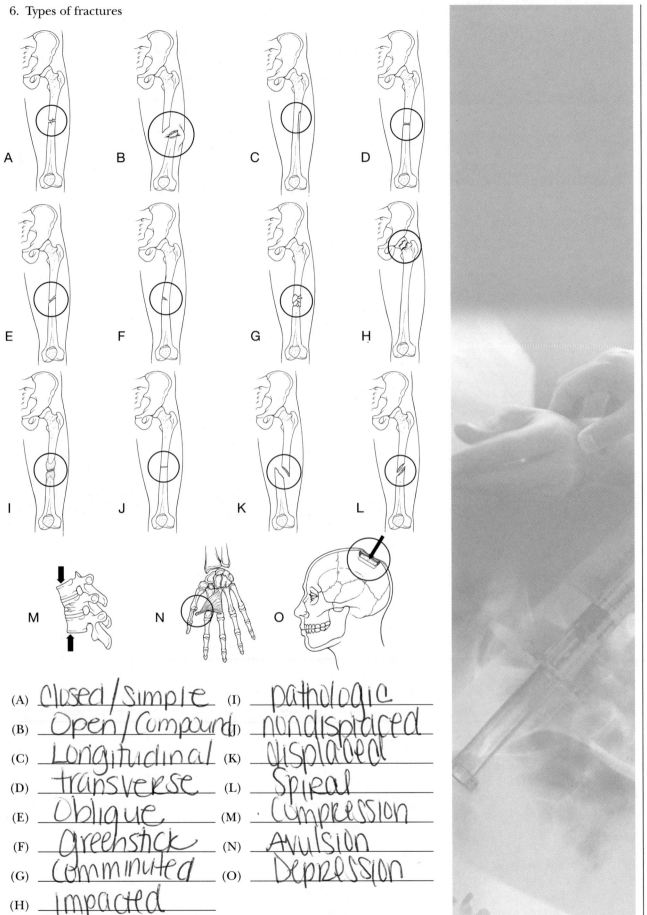

(A) Closed/simple
(B) Open/Compound
(C) Longitudinal
(D) transverse
(E) Oblique
(F) Greenstick
(G) Comminuted
(H) Impacted
(I) pathologic
(J) nondisplaced
(K) displaced
(L) Spiral
(M) Compression
(N) Avulsion
(O) Depression

Copyright ©2004, Elsevier. All rights reserved.

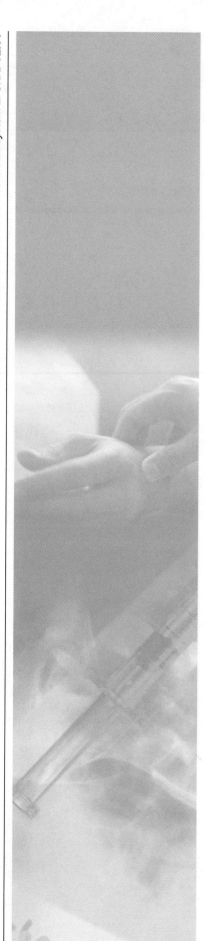

# PATIENT SCREENING

*For each scenario that follows, explain how and why you would schedule an appointment or suggest a referral based on the patient's reported symptoms.* **First, review the "Guidelines for Patient Screening Exercises" found on page iv in the "Introduction."**

1. The mother of a 12-year-old girl calls in saying her daughter has started complaining of back pain and fatigue. She also states that she has noticed her daughter's skirts do not hang evenly and that the school nurse has suggested an examination for scoliosis. How do you handle this phone call?

   _____

   _____

   _____

2. A patient calls in asking for an appointment saying that he has a red, itchy rash with a red circle center resembling the bull's eye on a target (target lesion) on his arm. He tells you he was out in the woods 2 days ago and thinks that a tick bit him. He thinks that the physician should see him. How do you respond to this call?

   _____

   _____

   _____

3. A male patient calls in telling you that he is experiencing severe, almost excruciating pain in the first joint of his left great toe. He has experienced this before and the pain usually will peak after several hours and then subside gradually. He also has a slight fever and chills. How do you respond to this call?

   _____

   _____

   _____

4. A patient calls the office saying he just twisted his ankle while walking up the stairs. He is complaining of localized pain and says he cannot stand on his leg. How do you handle this call?

   _____

   _____

   _____

5. A patient calls in saying while she was cutting a watermelon her knife slipped and she cut the middle finger on her left hand. The bleeding is controlled but she cannot bend her finger. The physician is gone from the office for the day. How do you handle this call?

   _____

   _____

   _____

Copyright ©2004, Elsevier. All rights reserved.

# PATIENT TEACHING

*For each scenario below, outline the appropriate patient teaching you would perform.*
***First, review the "Guidelines for Patient-Teaching Exercises" found on page iv in the "Introduction."***

1. **OSTEOARTHRITIS**

   An established patient with a history of osteoarthritis is undergoing on-going therapy, which includes drug therapy and a gentle exercise regimen. The patient is discouraged because of increased pain and loss of mobility. The physician instructs you to provide printed information regarding therapeutic diets and exercise for the patient. Additionally, you are to review intended effects of the prescribed drug therapy. How do you handle this patient-teaching opportunity?

   _____

   _____

   _____

   _____

   _____

2. **LYME DISEASE**

   A male patient has been diagnosed with Lyme disease. Antibiotic therapy has been prescribed. The patient has been told to return for a check-up in 1 week. The physician asks you to provide the patient with printed information concerning therapy that is advised in the treatment of this condition. How would you handle this patient-teaching opportunity?

   _____

   _____

   _____

   _____

   _____

3. **GOUT**

   An individual has been diagnosed with gout. The physician has instructed you to provide the patient with printed information regarding therapy for treatment of gout. How do you approach this patient-teaching opportunity?

   _____

   _____

   _____

   _____

   _____

Copyright ©2004, Elsevier. All rights reserved.

4. **OSTEOPOROSIS**

An older woman has been diagnosed with osteoporosis. The physician asks you to provide the patient with printed information concerning therapy that is advised in the treatment of this condition. How do you handle this patient-teaching opportunity?

_____

_____

_____

_____

_____

5. **FRACTURES**

An individual has a fracture of the ulna and radius at the wrist. A cast was placed on the area a few weeks earlier, and the patient is now requesting additional information about therapy for the hand, wrist, and arm. The physician has explained the anticipated therapy to the patient and requests you review this information with him or her. How do you handle this patient-teaching opportunity?

_____

_____

_____

_____

_____

# ESSAY QUESTION

*Write a response to the following question or statement. Use a separate sheet of paper if more space is needed.*

Describe the possible treatments for simple and compound fractures.

_____

_____

_____

_____

_____

_____

_____

_____

_____

_____

Copyright ©2004, Elsevier. All rights reserved.

# CERTIFICATION EXAMINATION REVIEW

*Circle the letter of the choice that best completes the statement or answers the question.*

1. Lordosis is a(an) _____ curvature of the spine.
   a. Lateral
   b. Inward (swayback)
   c. Outward
   d. None of the above

2. Scoliosis is a(an) _____ curvature of the spine.
   a. Lateral (sideways)
   b. Inward (swayback)
   c. Outward
   d. None of the above

3. Kyphosis is a(an) _____ curvature of the spine.
   a. Lateral
   b. Inward (swayback)
   c. Outward
   d. None of the above

4. Gouty arthritis is an inflammation of the joints caused by
   a. An excessive level of uric acid in the joints
   b. An excessive level of serum protein
   c. Streptococcus bacteria
   d. None of the above

5. A fracture with a break in the bone and a wound is a _____ fracture.
   a. Spiral
   b. Comminuted
   c. Compound, through the skin
   d. None of the above

6. A fracture with splintered or crushed bone is a
   a. Comminuted fracture
   b. Simple fracture
   c. Greenstick fracture
   d. None of the above

7. When a bone is fractured as a result of disease, it is called a _____ fracture.
   a. Greenstick
   b. Pathologic
   c. Spiral fracture
   d. None of the above

8. Atrophy is the wasting away or deterioration of a
   a. Bone
   b. Ligament
   c. Muscle
   d. None of the above

9. A severed tendon causes immediate and severe pain, inflammation, and
   a. Decreases mobility of the affected part
   b. Complete immobility of the affected part
   c. Weakness of the affected part
   d. None of the above

Copyright ©2004, Elsevier. All rights reserved.

10. Spurs are a common problem diagnosed in
    a. Individuals with bone deficiency
    b. Individuals active in sports, especially runners
    c. Individuals who use repetitive hand and wrist motions in their employment
    d. None of the above

11. Lyme disease is transmitted from a bacteria that is carried by a
    a. Mosquito
    b. Bee
    c. Tick
    d. All of the above

12. Tendons are tough strands or cords of dense connective tissue that attach muscle to
    a. Muscle
    b. Joints
    c. Bones
    d. None of the above

13. Collagen is a major supporting element or glue in
    a. Muscles
    b. Ligaments
    c. Connective tissue
    d. None of the above

14. The skeletal system is composed of _____ bones.
    a. 200
    b. 208
    c. 308
    d. None of the above

15. Osteomyelitis is a(an)
    a. Chronic progressive inflammatory disease
    b. Infection in a bone that can lead to abscess formation and sequestrum when not properly cared for
    c. Progressive weakening of the skeletal muscles
    d. None of the above

Copyright ©2004, Elsevier. All rights reserved.

# CHAPTER 8

# Diseases and Conditions of the Digestive System

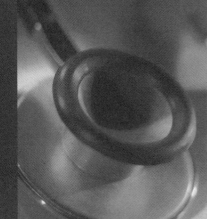

## WORD DEFINITIONS

*Define the following basic medical terms:*

1. Apicectomy — Surgical Removal of an anatomical apex

2. Cholinergic —

3. Colectomy — Excision of/part of the colon

4. Erosion — destruction if a surface area of tissue

5. Fissure — break or slit in tissue at the junction of skin + mucous membrane

6. Fistula — abnormal passage leading from an abscess/hollow organ to the body surface

7. Gangrene — local death of soft tissues due to loss of blood supply

8. Hematemesis — vomiting of blood

9. Leukoplakia —

10. Ligation — Surgical process by tying an anatomical caenna

11. Lymphadenopathy — abnormal enlargement of the lymph nodes

12. Malaise —

13. Metastasis —

14. Odynophagia — pain produced while swallowing

15. Pseudomembranous — presence or formation of a false membrane

16. Retrosternal — situated or occurring behind the sternum

17. Valsalva maneuver —

Copyright ©2004, Elsevier. All rights reserved.

# GLOSSARY TERMS

*Define the following chapter glossary terms:*

1. Anastomoses — Surgical connection between 2 vessels/ tubular structure
2. Aphthous ulcers — Recurrent painful canker sores in mouth
3. Cachexia — profound/marked wasting disorder
4. Diaphoretic — profuse perspiration
5. Fissures — crack/groove on a surface
6. Fistulas — abnormal tube-like passageway
7. Gangrene — death of tissue caused by a ↓ of blood
8. H2-receptor antagonist —
9. Hemostasis — condition of controlled bleeding
10. Hepatomegaly — enlargement of the liver
11. Hyperemic — excessive amount of blood in an area
12. Hypovolemic shock — blood in circulation system is decreased
13. Jaundiced — yellowing of the skin
14. Lavage — cleaning of a cavity w/ liquid
15. Malocclusion — improper positioning faulty contact of the teeth
16. Myalgia — muscle pain
17. Peritonitis — inflammation of lining of abdominal cavity
18. Proton pump inhibitor — drug that blocks gastric acid secretion
19. Reflux — backward flow
20. Stearrhea — presence of malabsorbed fat in the feces

# SHORT ANSWER

*Answer the following questions:*

1. Identify the function of the teeth.

2. List three reasons that a person may be missing permanent teeth.

Copyright ©2004, Elsevier. All rights reserved.

3. Describe how oral tumors begin.

_____

4. What symptom usually prompts a person to seek medical treatment for temporomandibular joint syndrome?

_____

5. Is thrush a bacterial, fungal, or viral infection?

_____

6. Cite statistics of incidence of squamous cell oral cancers.

_____

7. What lifestyle factors contribute to up to 80% of cases of oral cancer?

_____

_____

8. List treatment options for oral cancer.

_____

_____

9. Identify the main symptom that a patient experiences with esophagitis.

_____

10. Name the main cause of gastritis.

_____

11. Name the country with the highest incidence of gastric cancer in the world.

_____

12. Which sex has the highest occurrence of gastric cancer?

_____

13. Cite the length of the appendix.

_____

14. Identify the function of the appendix.

_____

15. Name the device that patients sometimes wear it they have a hernia.

_____

16. Identify the area of the alimentary canal that can be affected by Crohn disease.

_____

Copyright ©2004, Elsevier. All rights reserved.

17. Name the type of cancer that a patient with chronic ulcerative colitis is at risk to develop.

_____

18. Explain the goal of treatment for gastroenteritis.

_____

_____

19. List the symptoms and signs of intestinal obstruction.

_____

20. Which portion of the colon is usually the site of diverticulosis?

_____

21. Name the third most common site of cancer incidence and cause of death in both men and women.

_____

22. At what age should annual fecal occult testing begin for people at average risk for colorectal cancer?

_____

23. Can peritonitis be life threatening?

_____

24. In which sex is cirrhosis diagnosed more frequently?

_____

25. Identify the incubation period for hepatitis A.

_____

26. List the four fat-soluble vitamins that are stored in fat tissue.

_____

## FILL IN THE BLANKS

*Fill in the blanks with the correct terms. A Word List has been provided. Words used twice are indicated with a (2).*

1. The _alimentary canal_ processes and transports products of _digestion_.

2. The function of the teeth is _mastication_ to break down food into pieces that can be _swallowed_ and digested _easily_.

Copyright ©2004, Elsevier. All rights reserved.

3. Periodontitis, also called _____ disease, is destructive

   _____ and bone _____ around one

   or more of the _____.

4. A _____ _____ is a pus-filled sac

   that develops in the _____ surrounding the

   _____ of the root.

5. Herpes simplex blisters can develop on the ___**lips**___ and

   inside the ___**mouth**___, producing painful ___**ulcers**___

   that last a few hours or ___**days**___.

6. Oral cancer usually appears as a ___**white**___, patchy lesion

   or an ___**oral**___ ulcer that ___**fails**___ to

   heal.

7. Normal esophageal reflux can result from ___**overeating**___,

   pregnancy, or ___**weight**___ gain.

8. Treatment of esophagitis includes several weeks of a

   ___**bland**___ ___**diet**___ to calm the

   ___**inflammation**___ and the use of ___**strong**___ antacids.

9. A ___**hiatal**___ hernia exists when the ___**upper**___

   part of the ___**stomach**___ protrudes through the

   ___**esophageal**___ opening of the diaphragm into the thoracic cavity.

10. A _____ is a mechanical bowel obstruction where

    there is a twisting of the bowel on itself.

11. Short-bowel ___**syndrome**___ is the result of an

    ___**insufficient**___ amount of functioning small bowel to

    ___**absorb**___ nutrients, fluid, ___**vitamins**___, and

    minerals that the body needs.

12. Hemorrhoids are ___**varicose**___ dilations of a vein in the

    ___**anal**___ ___**canal**___ or the anorectal area.

13. Some early liver _____ can be reversed. Chronic

    _____ hepatic disease is the _____

    leading cause of death in the United States.

Copyright ©2004, Elsevier. All rights reserved.

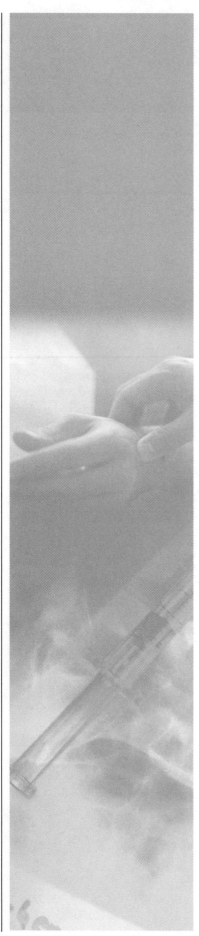

14. Celiac disease is a disease of the _small intestine_ that is characterized by _malabsorption gluten intolerance_ and _damage_ to the lining of the intestine.

## WORD LIST

absorb, alimentary canal, anal canal, base, bland diet, bone, damage (2), days, digestion, easily, eleventh, esophageal, fails, gluten intolerance, gum, heal, hiatal, inflammation, insufficient, lips, malabsorption, mastication, mouth, oral, overeating, periodontal, progressive, small intestine, stomach, strong, swallowed, syndrome, teeth, tissue, tooth abscess, ulcers, upper, varicose, vitamins, volvulus, weight, white

# ANATOMIC STRUCTURES

*Identify the following structures of the digestive system and their functions.*

1. Main and accessory organs of the normal digestive system

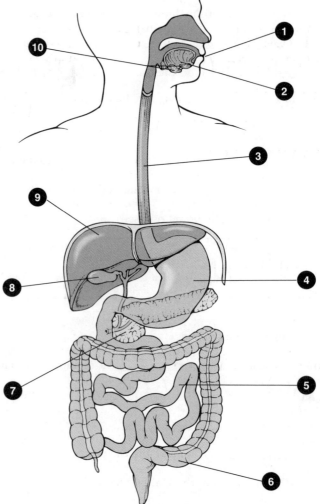

**Accessory Organs**          **Main Organs**

Copyright ©2004, Elsevier. All rights reserved.

(1) mouth: chewing food; initial carb. digestion
(2) pharynx: swallowing
(3) esophagus: transport food 2 stomach; secretion of mucus
(4) stomach: churning of food
(5) small intestine: final digestion of gastric juice
(6) large intestine: elimination of wastes
(7) pancreas: release of pancreatic juice into duodenum 2 digest
(8) gallbladder: release of bile
(9) liver: manufacture bile
(10) salivary glands: secretion of saliva

## PATIENT SCREENING

*For each scenario below, explain how and why you would schedule an appointment or suggest a referral based on the patient's reported symptoms.* **First, review the "Guidelines for Patient-Screening Exercises" found on page iv in the "Introduction."**

1. A male patient calls stating he is experiencing pain in the "jaw joint" on the right side of his mouth. He says he has been hearing a clicking sound when he chews and the pain is getting progressively worse. He also says he is having problems opening his mouth. He requests an appointment to see the physician. How do you handle this phone call?

_____

_____

_____

2. A patient calls stating he is experiencing "heartburn," usually most severe at night. He also says he has episodes of belching causing a burning sensation in his mouth and chest. How do you handle this phone call?

_____

_____

_____

3. The father of a 16-year-old adolescent calls the office stating his son is experiencing abdominal pain that started as vague discomfort around the navel. Now a few hours later, it has localized in the right lower quadrant. He has just become nauseated and has a slight fever. How do you handle this call?

_____

_____

_____

Copyright ©2004, Elsevier. All rights reserved.

4. A patient calls stating she is experiencing pain in the right upper quadrant of the abdomen, often radiating to the right upper back in the area of the scapula. Nausea and vomiting accompany the pain. She thinks her skin is turning yellow. How do you respond to this call?

_____

_____

_____

5. The mother of a 16-year-old adolescent calls in advising she wants her daughter to be seen by the physician. The girl is refusing to eat and is preoccupied with obesity and obsessed with her weight. Although she experiences continued weight loss, she does not believe anything is wrong. How do you handle this phone call?

_____

_____

_____

# PATIENT TEACHING

*For each scenario below, outline the appropriate patient teaching you would perform.*
**First, review the "Guidelines for Patient-Teaching Exercises" found on page iv in the "Introduction."**

1. **DENTAL CARIES**
A patient is noted to be in need of dental assessment. The physician suggests that until a dental appointment can be made and kept, the patient should be instructed on proper oral hygiene and dental care. How do you handle this patient-teaching opportunity?

_____

_____

_____

2. **HERPES SIMPLEX**
A patient has a large "cold sore" on the upper lip that is quite painful. It is diagnosed as a herpes simplex eruption. You are instructed to provide printed information regarding the care of the eruption and ways to avoid spreading this contagious lesion. How do you approach this patient-teaching opportunity?

_____

_____

_____

_____

Copyright ©2004, Elsevier. All rights reserved.

3. **GASTROESOPHAGEAL REFLUX DISORDER**

An individual experiencing gastroesophageal reflux disorder (GERD) requires instructions about methods to avoid the reflux. The physician requests you to provide him or her with printed information and to explain how he or she can lessen the occurrence of the attacks. How do you approach this patient-teaching opportunity?

_____

_____

_____

_____

_____

_____

4. **PEPTIC ULCERS**

An individual has been diagnosed with a peptic ulcer. The physician requests you reinforce his instructions to the patient by using printed material available in the office. How do you approach this patient-teaching opportunity?

_____

_____

_____

_____

_____

_____

5. **CHOLECYSTITIS**

An individual has been experiencing severe right-sided epigastric pain after eating. The diagnosis of cholecystitis has been made. The physician requests you reinforce her dietary instructions to the patient using printed dietary information available in the office. How do you approach this patient-teaching opportunity?

_____

_____

_____

_____

_____

_____

Copyright ©2004, Elsevier. All rights reserved.

# ESSAY QUESTION

*Write a response to the following question or statement. Use a separate sheet of paper if more space is needed.*

Describe the signs and symptoms that are associated with Crohn disease and available options for treatment.

_____

_____

_____

_____

_____

_____

_____

_____

_____

_____

_____

_____

_____

_____

_____

_____

_____

_____

_____

# CERTIFICATION EXAMINATION REVIEW

*Circle the letter of the choice that best completes the statement or answers the question.*

1. The transmission route for _____ is fecal oral and is transmitted by contaminated water, food, and stools. Poor hygiene also plays a role in the transmission.
   a. Hepatitis A
   b. Hepatitis B
   c. Hepatitis C
   d. None of the above

Copyright ©2004, Elsevier. All rights reserved.

2. The use of broad-spectrum antibiotics is associated with the occurrence of
   a. Esophagitis
   b. Gastritis
   c. Pseudomembranous enterocolitis
   d. None of the above

3. The symptoms of biliary colic with radiating pain and jaundice accompany
   a. Appendicitis
   b. Cholecystitis
   c. Cholelithiasis
   d. All of the above

4. Anorexia nervosa is an eating disorder in which the person perceives their body image as
   a. Thin
   b. Just right
   c. Overweight
   d. None of the above

5. A chronic irreversible degeneration of the liver is
   a. Cholecystitis
   b. Pancreatitis
   c. Cholelithiasis
   d. Cirrhosis

6. The route of transmission for _____ is by blood or body fluid.
   a. Hepatitis A
   b. Hepatitis B
   c. Hepatitis C
   d. Both b and c

7. Peritonitis is an infection that involves the
   a. Liver
   b. Serous membrane that lines the abdominal cavity
   c. Pancreas
   d. None of the above

8. Neoplasm, volvulus, intussusception, and fecal impaction can all cause
   a. Diverticulitis
   b. Diverticulosis
   c. Mechanical bowel obstruction
   d. None of the above

9. The fourth leading cause of cancer-related death in the United States is
   a. Colon cancer
   b. Gastric cancer
   c. Pancreatic cancer
   d. None of the above

10. Allergic reaction or irritation from foods, mechanical injury, medications, poisons, alcohol, and infectious diseases may damage the gastric lining and cause
    a. Diverticulitis
    b. Gastritis
    c. Hepatitis
    d. None of the above

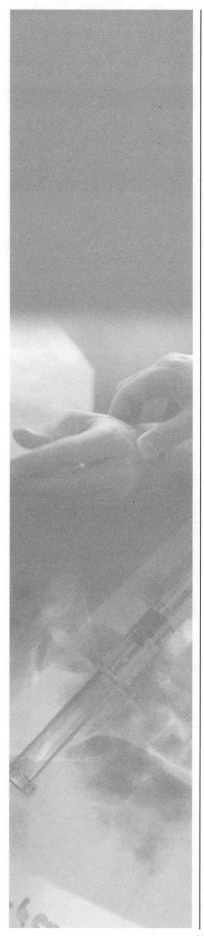

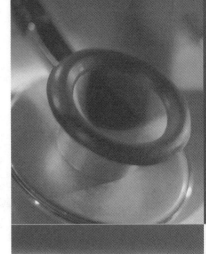

# CHAPTER 9

# Diseases and Conditions of the Respiratory System

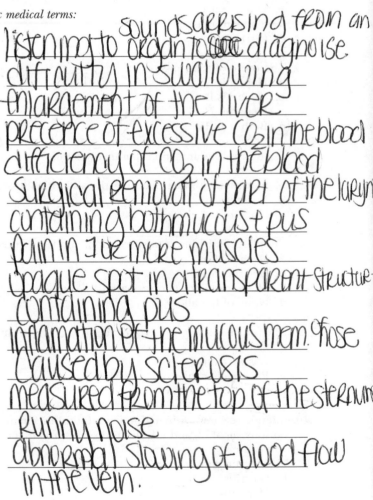

## WORD DEFINITIONS

*Define the following basic medical terms:*

1. Auscultation — listening to sounds arising from an organ to make diagnoise.

2. Dysphagia — difficulty in swallowing

3. Hepatomegaly — enlargement of the liver

4. Hypercapnia — presence of excessive $CO_2$ in the blood

5. Hypocapnia — difficiency of $CO_2$ in the blood

6. Laryngectomy — surgical removal of part of the laryn

7. Mucopurulent — containing both mucous + pus

8. Myalgia — pain in 1 or more muscles

9. Opacities — opaque spot in a transparent structure

10. Purulent — containing pus

11. Rhinitis — inflamation of the mucous mem. of nose

12. Sclerosing — caused by sclerosis

13. Suprasternal — measured from the top of the sternum

14. Tinnitus — runny noise

15. Venostasis — abnormal slowing of blood flow in the vein.

Copyright ©2004, Elsevier. All rights reserved.

# GLOSSARY TERMS

*Define the following chapter glossary terms:*

1. Agranulocytosis — (decrease) Sudden ↓ in the the # of wbc
2. Aphonia — inability to produce normal speech sounds or loss of voice
3. Bifurcates — split into 2 branches
4. Cephalgia — headache; pain in the head
5. Coagulation — process of clot formation
6. Cyanosis — bluish appearance of the skin/mucous membrane
7. Emboli — a mass that causes a blocked artery
8. Epistaxis — bleeding from the nose
9. Exsanguination — excessive loss of blood from a part
10. Insidious — refers to the onset of a disease w/o symptoms
11. Mediastinum — area in the chest between the lungs
12. Mycoplasma — microscopic organism that lacks rigid cell walls
13. Perfusion — delivery of O₂ & other nutrients to the tissue by the blood
14. Rales — abnormal crackling sound made by the lungs during inspiration
15. Rhonchi —
16. Stenosis — narrowing of an opening
17. Stridor — ↑ pitched breathing sound caused by obstruction of a air passageway, this under breathing
18. Substernal retraction — chest wall under the sternum
19. Tachypnea — rapid heart rate ↑ 100 bpm
20. Thoracentesis — surgical puncture into the thoracic cavity to remove accumulated fluid/air

# SHORT ANSWER

*Answer the following questions:*

1. Name the primary function of the lungs.

   Respiration

2. Identify the dome-shaped muscle that assists with respiration.

   diaphragm

Copyright ©2004, Elsevier. All rights reserved.

3. What are two causes for respiratory failure?

*smoking / fluid in lungs*

4. Does an antibiotic effectively treat a common cold?

*no*

5. Identify the cause of sinusitis.

*allergies, bacterial infection*

6. What is unique about nasopharyngeal carcinoma?

*neck pain - common pain*

7. Name the most common symptom of nasopharyngeal carcinoma that is reported in over 90% of patients who are diagnosed with this type of cancer.

8. Identify the condition that causes narrowing and obstruction of the air passage, making breathing more difficult.

*deviated septum*

9. Do nasal polyps tend to recur after surgical removal?

*yes*

10. Are nosebleeds more common in children or adults?

*children*

11. Identify the type of carcinoma that is the cause of most laryngeal neoplasms.

12. Identify what occurs when a clot of foreign material lodges in and occludes an artery in the pulmonary circulation.

*pulmonery embolism*

13. Name the drug of choice used to treat most pulmonary emboli.

*heppin, thrombic literal drugs*

14. Identify the age groups at most risk for respiratory syncytial viral (RSV) infection.

*(x3) young children / elderly / ppl. w/HIV*

15. Name the antifungal medicine used to treat histoplasmosis.

*intatelison B*

16. What does the term pneumoconiosis mean?

*death in the lungs*
*dust*

Copyright ©2004, Elsevier. All rights reserved.

17. Name the condition that causes sharp needlelike pain and increases with inspiration and coughing.

_closidc/predisidu—wet/dry_

18. Identify the two types of pleurisy.

_wet/dry_

19. What accumulates in the pleural cavity when hemothorax is the diagnosis?

_blood/fluid_

20. Describe the fracture that occurs when the patient is diagnosed with flail chest.

_3 ribs fractured in 2 different places_

21. Identify the intradermal test that is used to detect the presence of tuberculin antibodies.

_ppd_

22. Is the prognosis for adult respiratory distress syndrome good or poor?

_poor_

23. Name the primary risk factor for developing lung cancer.

_smoking_

24. What is the cause of severe acute respiratory syndrome (SARS)?

_coronal viruse_

25. Identify the drug of choice to treat pneumococcal pneumonia.

_penasilin_

## FILL IN THE BLANKS

*Fill in the blanks with the correct terms. A Word List has been provided. Words used twice are indicated with a (2).*

1. In the lungs, _oxygen_ inhaled from the air is _exchanged_ with _carbon_ _dioxide_ from the blood; this process is called _external_ respiration.

2. On inspiration, the diaphragm _contracts_, pulling downward and causing air to be _sucked_ _into_ the lungs. During expiration, the diaphragm _relaxes_, pushing _upward_ and forcing air _out_ of the lungs.

Copyright ©2004, Elsevier. All rights reserved.

3. An ordinary cold should clear up in ____4____ to ____5____ days.

4. General _____ health _____

one to the common cold.

5. The sinuses, _____ in the bones lying

_____ the nose, are normally ____air____

filled.

6. Because the opening of the larynx is _____,

inflammation of the larynx sometimes _____

with _____.

7. Hemorrhage from the nose, known as _____, is a

common _____ emergency.

8. The larynx plays an important role in _____,

swallowing, _____, and protection of the

_____ airway.

9. Trauma, _____ of a _____,

or _____ can cause bronchial bleeding, as can

bronchitis or bronchiectasis.

10. Atelectasis follows incomplete _____ of the lobules

or _____ of the _____, with

partial or complete _____ of the lung.

11. Respiratory syncytial virus has the greatest occurrence during the

_____ months.

12. Possible complications of influenza are _____,

sinusitis, _____ _____, and

cervical _____.

13. Collapse of a lung causes severe _____ of

_____, sudden sharp _____

_____, falling _____

_____, rapid _____ pulse,

and _____ and weak _____.

Copyright ©2004, Elsevier. All rights reserved.

14. The treatment for hemothorax includes re-expanding the lung, usually

by _____ with closed _____

to evacuate the blood.

15. Pulmonary tuberculosis is acquired by the _____

of a _____ droplet _____

that contains the _____ _____.

## WORD LIST

4, 5, air, behind, blood pressure, breath, breathing, bronchitis, calcification, carbon dioxide, cavities, chest pain, collapse, contracts, drainage, dried, epistaxis, erosion, exchanged, expansion, external, inhalation, interferes, lower, lungs, lymphadenopathy, narrow, nucleus, otitis media, out, oxygen, predisposes, poor, relaxes, respiration (2), segments, shallow, shortness, speech, sucked into, sudden, thoracentesis, tubercle bacillus, tumors, upward, vessel, weak, winter

## ANATOMIC STRUCTURES

*Identify the structures in the following anatomic diagrams.*

1. Normal lower respiratory system

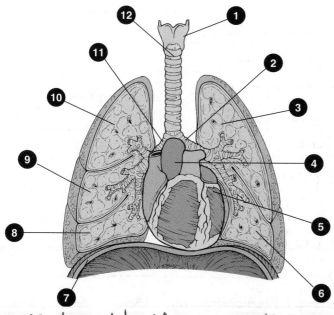

(1) _thyroid cartilage_    (7) _diaphragm_

(2) _left bronchus_    (8) _right lower lobe_

(3) _left upper lobe_    (9) _right middle lobe_

(4) _aorta_    (10) _right upper lobe_

(5) _heart_    (11) _right bronchus_

(6) _left lower lobe_    (12) _trachea_

Copyright ©2004, Elsevier. All rights reserved.

2. Normal upper respiratory system

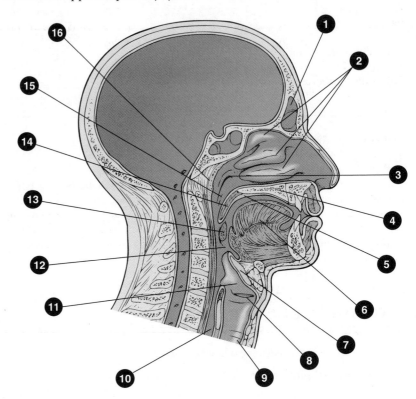

(1) Frontal Sinus

(2) Turbinates

(3) Office of eustachian tube

(4) hard palate

(5) Soft palate

(6) tongue

(7) Epiglottis

(8) Vocal cords

(9) Trachea

(10) Esophagus

(11) Larynx

(12) Oropharynx

(13) palatine tonsil

(14) Uvula

(15) nasopharynx

(16) pharyngeal tonsil

Copyright ©2004, Elsevier. All rights reserved.

# PATIENT SCREENING

*For each scenario that follows, explain how and why you would schedule an appointment or suggest a referral based on the patient's reported symptoms.* **First, review the "Guidelines for Patient-Screening Exercises" found on page iv in the "Introduction."**

1. A male patient calls in reporting he is experiencing headache over both eyes, especially on waking up in the morning. He also says there is pain and tenderness above the eyes, which occurs when bending over. Additionally, he reports a thick, greenish yellow drainage and has a slight temperature. How do you handle this phone call?

_____

_____

_____

_____

_____

2. A female patient calls in saying she is experiencing hoarseness, difficulty talking, a slight fever, and a sore throat. How do you respond to this call?

_____

_____

_____

_____

_____

3. A wife calls in saying her husband is experiencing a severe nosebleed. The nose has been bleeding for about 20 minutes, and they cannot get it to stop. How do you handle this phone call?

_____

_____

_____

_____

_____

4. A male patient calls in saying he is coughing and spitting up blood. How do you respond to this call?

_____

_____

_____

_____

_____

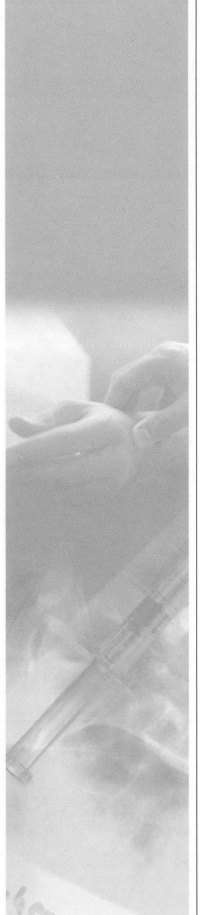

Copyright ©2004, Elsevier. All rights reserved.

5. A female patient calls in and advises that she is experiencing a deep, persistent, productive cough. She has thick, yellow-to-gray sputum. Additionally, she reports shortness of breath, wheezing, a slightly elevated temperature, and pain in the upper chest, which is aggravated by the cough. How do you respond to this call?

_____

_____

_____

_____

_____

## PATIENT TEACHING

*For each scenario below, outline the appropriate patient teaching you would perform.*
***First, review the "Guidelines for Patient-Teaching Exercises" found on page iv in the "Introduction."***

1. **PHARYNGITIS**
   A patient has been diagnosed with recurrent pharyngitis. A course of antibiotic therapy has been prescribed. The physician has printed information regarding comfort measures. You are asked to provide the patient with the list, as well as encourage compliance with completing the antibiotic regimen. How do you approach this patient-teaching opportunity?

   _____

   _____

   _____

   _____

   _____

2. **LARYNGITIS**
   Recurring laryngitis has been diagnosed for a patient who can hardly speak. The physician instructs you to explain the importance of completing the antibiotic regimen. The office has printed instructions for the patient, and you are expected to provide the patient with the list and explain any areas not fully understood. How do you approach this patient-teaching opportunity?

   _____

   _____

   _____

   _____

   _____

Copyright ©2004, Elsevier. All rights reserved.

3. **EPISTAXIS**

   A child has experienced recurring nosebleeds in the past few months. The parents are becoming apprehensive about them, and the physician asks you to reinforce his instructions to the parents by providing them with written information concerning epistaxis. How do you approach this patient-teaching opportunity?

   _____

   _____

   _____

   _____

   _____

4. **PNEUMOCONIOSIS**

   A patient has been diagnosed with pneumoconiosis. Along with the use of corticosteroid drugs, treatment is to include bronchodilators, oxygen therapy, and chest physical therapy to help remove secretions. How do you approach this patient-teaching opportunity?

   _____

   _____

   _____

   _____

   _____

5. **INFLUENZA**

   An individual is experiencing flulike symptoms. After being seen by the physician, the patient is diagnosed with influenza. The physician requests you to provide the patient with the printed patient-teaching instructions. How do you approach this patient-teaching opportunity?

   _____

   _____

   _____

   _____

   _____

Copyright ©2004, Elsevier. All rights reserved.

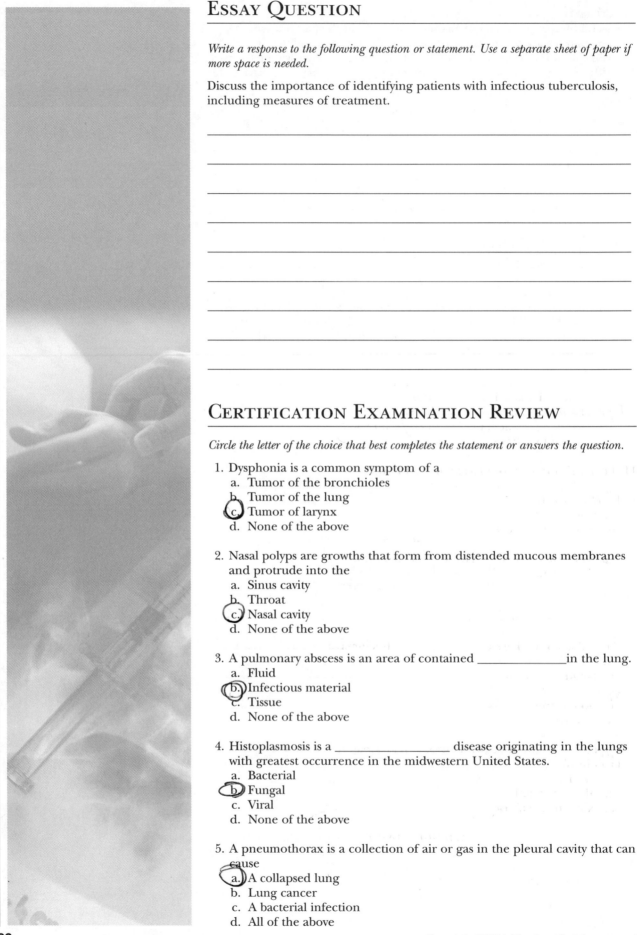

# ESSAY QUESTION

*Write a response to the following question or statement. Use a separate sheet of paper if more space is needed.*

Discuss the importance of identifying patients with infectious tuberculosis, including measures of treatment.

_____

_____

_____

_____

_____

_____

_____

_____

# CERTIFICATION EXAMINATION REVIEW

*Circle the letter of the choice that best completes the statement or answers the question.*

1. Dysphonia is a common symptom of a
   a. Tumor of the bronchioles
   b. Tumor of the lung
   c. Tumor of larynx
   d. None of the above

2. Nasal polyps are growths that form from distended mucous membranes and protrude into the
   a. Sinus cavity
   b. Throat
   c. Nasal cavity
   d. None of the above

3. A pulmonary abscess is an area of contained _____ in the lung.
   a. Fluid
   b. Infectious material
   c. Tissue
   d. None of the above

4. Histoplasmosis is a _____ disease originating in the lungs with greatest occurrence in the midwestern United States.
   a. Bacterial
   b. Fungal
   c. Viral
   d. None of the above

5. A pneumothorax is a collection of air or gas in the pleural cavity that can cause
   a. A collapsed lung
   b. Lung cancer
   c. A bacterial infection
   d. All of the above

Copyright ©2004, Elsevier. All rights reserved.

6. Infectious mononucleosis is caused from
   a. Epstein-Barr Virus
   b. Histoplasmosis
   c. Bacteria
   d. None of the above

7. Organism specific antibiotics are used to treat
   a. Histoplasmosis
   b. Mononucleosis
   c. Bacterial pneumonia
   d. All of the above

8. Exposure to _____ smoke may make an individual more susceptible to any respiratory condition.
   a. Primary
   b. Secondary
   c. Both a and b
   d. None of the above

9. Pneumoconiosis is caused from inhalation of
   a. An airborne virus
   b. Moisture droplets
   c. Inorganic dust
   d. All of the above

10. Examples of occupational diseases include
    a. Pneumonia, sinusitis, and rhinitis
    b. Asbestosis, anthracosis, and silicosis
    c. Flail chest, pulmonary abscess, and emphysema
    d. None of the above

11. Legionellosis is a more severe form of Pontiac fever, and both forms are
    a. Contagious
    b. Not contagious
    c. Congenital
    d. None of the above

12. Barrel chest, chronic cough, and dyspnea are all symptoms of
    a. Emphysema
    b. Pneumonia
    c. Hemothorax
    d. None of the above

13. With flail chest, there are _____ fractures of three or more adjacent ribs.
    a. Single
    b. Double
    c. Both a and b
    d. Neither a or b

14. Sinusotomy, antibiotics, and decongestants may all be treatments for
    a. Sinusitis
    b. Bronchitis
    c. Allergic rhinitis
    d. None of the above

15. There are almost 200 different viruses that are responsible for causing
    a. Sinusitis
    b. Bronchitis
    c. The common cold
    d. None of the above

Copyright ©2004, Elsevier. All rights reserved.

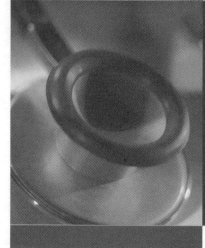

# CHAPTER 10

# Diseases and Conditions of the Circulatory System

## WORD DEFINITIONS

*Define the following basic medical terms:*

1. Anticoagulant

2. Antipyretic

3. Arteritis

4. Atheroma

5. Bronchodilator

6. Carditis

7. Endocarditis

8. ESR

9. Gingival

10. Hyperlipidemia

11. Leukocytosis

12. Polyarthritis

13. Polycythemia

14. Serous

15. Transdermal

preventing, Removing, allaying fever

inflamation arterial

abnormal fatty deposit in an artery

causing expansion of the bronchial air passage

inflamation of the ♥ muscle

inflamation of the lining of the ♥ & valves

presence of excess fat / lipids in the blood

↑ number in leukocytosis circulating in the blood

arthritis involving 2 or more joints

abnormal ↑ in the # of RBC circulating

resembling serum / having a thin watery constitution

supplying medication in a form for absorption through the skin into the bloodstream.

Copyright ©2004, Elsevier. All rights reserved.

# GLOSSARY TERMS

*Define the following chapter glossary terms:*

1. Aggregation — coming together of entities such as blood cells

2. Anaphylaxis — severe systemic allergic response characterized by redness, itching, swelling & water buildup

3. Angina pectoris

4. Angiotensin-converting enzyme — found on the surface of blood vessels in the lungs and other tissues w/ vasopressive action

5. Antibodies — immunoglobulin that may combine with a specific antigen to destroy or control it.

6. Arrhythmias — variation/loss of normal rythm of the heartbeat

7. Blood gas

8. Bruit — abnormal sound heard in auscultation

9. Collateral — small side branch of a blood vessel or nerve

10. Commissurotomy

11. Diuretics — increased formation & excretion of urine

12. Doppler — ultrasound technique, used to evaluate blood flow velocity

13. Gangrene — death of tissue caused by a ↓ /absence of blood supply

14. Hematocrit — % of total blood volume consisting of erythrocytes

15. Idiopathic — refers to a disease w/o a known/recognizable cause

16. Opacity — state of being opaque or not transparent

17. Perfusion — delivery of oxygen / other nutrients to the tissue by the blood.

18. Petechiae — tiny spider like hemorrhage under the skin

19. Plaque — deposit of hardened material lining the blood vessel

20. Prophylactic — prevention of disease

21. Purpura — discoloration of the skin caused by multiple min. hemorrages in the skin

22. Rales — abnormal crackling sound made by the lungs during inspiration

23. Sclerosing — hardening of a body part

24. Syncope — fainting, lightheadedness

25. Tamponade — compression of a part by pressure / collection of fluid

Copyright ©2004, Elsevier. All rights reserved.

## SHORT ANSWER

*Answer the following questions:*

1. The heart pumps how many quarts of blood throughout the body each minute?

   *5 quarts*

2. Identify the first symptom of coronary artery disease.

   *pain of the angina pectoris*

3. List individuals having the potential to be at increased risk for coronary artery disease.

   *40 yrs plus; men; white people; postmenopausel) women*

4. What is the experimental gene therapy that is being used to stimulate new growth of blood vessels for patients with coronary artery disease (CAD)?

   *Angioplasty*

5. Describe the pain that is experienced by a patient experiencing angina pectoris.

   *chest pain after exertion*

6. Identify the form of nitroglycerin that is helpful in preventing angina.

7. Cite the percentage of deaths occurring in the first hour after a myocardial infarction.

   *65%*

8. What measures are initiated to try to reverse cardiac arrest?

9. Name the most prevalent cardiovascular disorder in the United States.

10. List the symptoms of essential hypertension.

    *headaches, epistaxis, lightheadedness, syncope.*

11. Are people always aware they have hypertension?

    *NO*

12. Identify the cardiac test that helps in evaluating cardiac chamber size, ventricular function, and disease of the myocardium, valves, cardiac strictures, and pericardium.

Copyright ©2004, Elsevier. All rights reserved.

13. Cor pulmonale affects which side of the heart?

_right_

14. Describe the skin of a person with pulmonary edema.

_Skin becomes cold and clammy_

15. What type of growths on the cardiac valves characterizes endocarditis?

_inflamation on of the lining & the valves of the ♡_

16. Identify a preventative measure before dental work for people with endocarditis.

_____

17. Which valves of the heart can be affected by valvular heart disease?

_any of the 4 valves of the ♡_

18. Identify the cause of rheumatic heart disease.

_____

_____

19. Name the final option to treat rheumatic heart disease.

_____

20. List the symptoms associated with mitral valve prolapse.

_____

_____

21. How are cardiac arrhythmias diagnosed?

_Clinical picture a history of a traumatic event_

22. Which part of the heart fails to work effectively during cardiogenic shock?

_____

23. Explain the cause of cardiac tamponade.

_____

_____

24. List the three forms of arteriosclerosis.

_monckeberg, arteriusclerosis, arteri atherosclerosis_

25. Which form of arteriosclerosis is responsible for most myocardial and cerebral infarctions?

_____

Copyright ©2004, Elsevier. All rights reserved.

26. List the components of blood.

RBC, WBC, platelets, plasma

27. What causes hemolytic anemia?

28. How are leukemias classified?

cell type; degree of differentiation of the neoplastic cells

29. Name the form of leukemia that is the most common adult leukemia and accounts for 20% of childhood leukemias.

Acute Myelogenous Leukemia

30. Identify the initial symptoms of Hodgkin's disease.

painless enlargement of the lymph nodes in the neck or mediastineum

## FILL IN THE BLANKS

*Fill in the blanks with the correct terms. A Word List has been provided. Words used twice are indicated with a (2).*

1. The two upper chambers of the heart are called __atria__,

   and the two lower chambers are called __ventricles__.

2. Cardiac muscle tissue is composed of __striated__ __muscle__ __cells__.

3. Myocardial infarction results from insufficient __oxygen__ __supply__, as when a coronary __artery__ is occluded by atherosclerotic plaque, __thrombus__, or myocardial __muscle__ spasm.

4. Cardiopulmonary resuscitation (CPR) must be instituted within __4__ to __6__ minutes of the __cardiac__ arrest.

5. Elevated __blood__ __pressure__ __readings__ are the __first__ indication of hypertension.

Copyright ©2004, Elsevier. All rights reserved.

6. Pulmonary edema causes patients to experience __dyspnea__ and __coughing__, orthopnea, __increased__ cardiac and respiratory __rates__, and often __bloody__ frothy sputum.

7. Endocarditis is usually secondary to __bacteria__ in the blood stream.

8. Almost one third of all deaths in western countries are attributed to __heart__ __disease__.

9. Deposits of fat-containing substances called __plaque__ on the __lumen__ of the coronary arteries result in atherosclerosis.

10. Angioplasty is attempted to open up a constricted __artery__ in coronary artery disease.

11. Pulmonary edema is a condition of __fluid__ shift into the __extravascular__ spaces of the lungs.

12. Cardiomyopathy causes the patient to experience symptoms of __CHF__, including __dyspnea__, __fatigue__, __tachycardia__, __palpitations__, and occasionally __chest__ pain.

13. Myocarditis is frequently a __viral__, bacterial, __fungal__, or protozoal infection or complication of other diseases.

14. Valvular heart disease can occur in the form of __insufficiency__ or __stenosis__.

15. Arrhythmias occur when there is __interference__ with the __conduction__ system of the heart, resulting in an __abnormality__ of the heartbeat.

## WORD LIST

4, 6, abnormality, artery (2), atria, bacteria, blood pressure readings, bloody, cardiac, chest, congestive heart failure (CHF), conduction, coughing, dyspnea (2), extravascular, fatigue, first, fluid, fungal, heart disease, increased, insufficiency, interference, lumen, muscle, oxygen supply, palpitations, plaque, rates, stenosis, striated muscle cells, tachycardia, thrombus, ventricles, viral

Copyright ©2004, Elsevier. All rights reserved.

# ANATOMIC STRUCTURES

*Identify the structures in the following anatomic diagrams. For number 4, identify what occurs with each phase of the cardiac cycle.*

1. Anterior view of the heart and great vessels

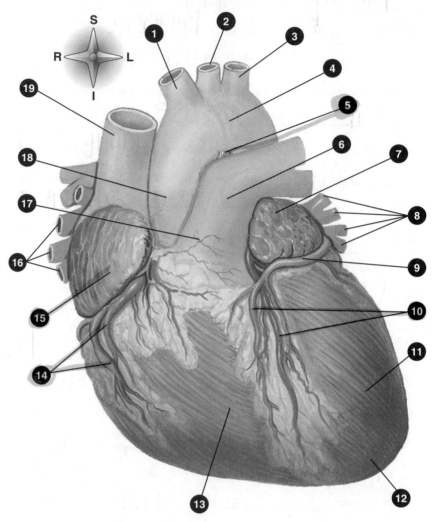

(1) Brachiocephalic trunk

(2) left common carotid artery

(3) left subclavian artery

(4) Arch of Aorta

(5) _____

(6) pulmonary trunk

(7) Auricle of left atrium

(8) left pulmonary veins

(9) great cardiac vein

(10) _____

(11) left ventricle

(12) Apex

(13) Right ventricle

(14) _____

(15) _____

(16) Right pulmonary veins

(17) conus arteriosus

(18) Ascending colon

(19) Superior vena cava

Copyright ©2004, Elsevier. All rights reserved.

2. Posterior view of the heart and great vessels

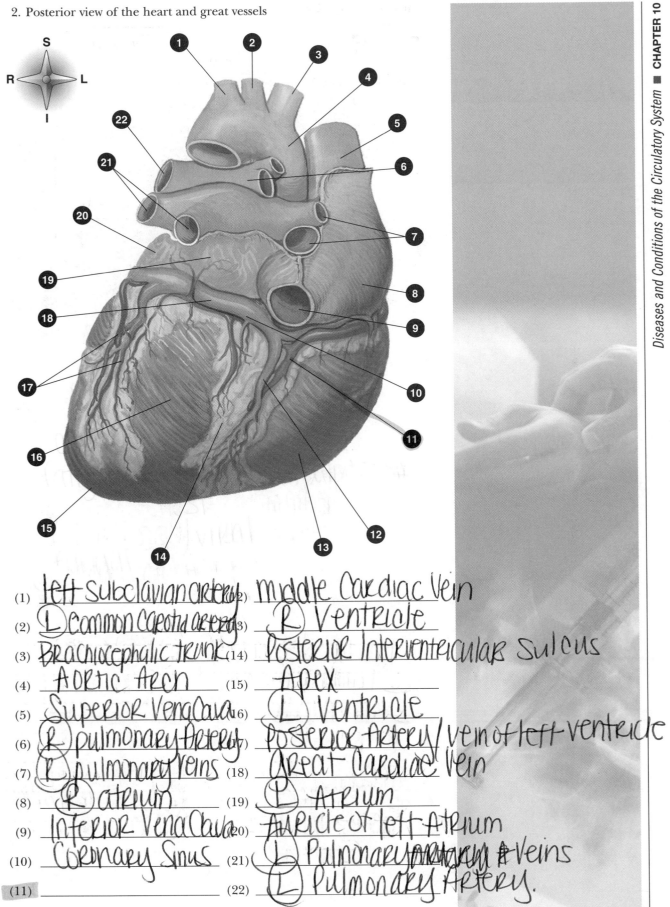

(1) left Subclavian artery
(2) L common carotid artery
(3) Brachiocephalic trunk
(4) Aortic Arch
(5) Superior Vena Cava
(6) R pulmonary Artery
(7) L pulmonary Veins
(8) R atrium
(9) Inferior Vena Cava
(10) Coronary Sinus
(11) _____

(12) Middle Cardiac Vein
(13) R Ventricle
(14) Posterior Interventricular Sulcus
(15) Apex
(16) L Ventricle
(17) Posterior Artery/vein of left ventricle
(18) great Cardiac Vein
(19) L Atrium
(20) Auricle of left Atrium
(21) L Pulmonary artery & Veins
(22) L pulmonary Artery.

Copyright ©2004, Elsevier. All rights reserved.

3. Circulation through the heart

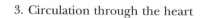

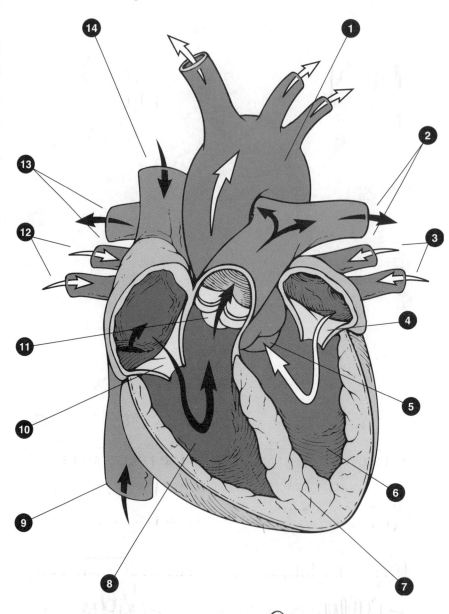

(1) ___Aorta___

(2) ___(L) Pulmonary Arteries___

(3) ___(L) Pulmonary Veins___

(4) ___Mitral Valve___

(5) ___Aortic Valve___

(6) ___(L) Ventricle___

(7) ___Interventricular Septum___

(8) ___(R) Ventricle___

(9) ___Inferior Vena Cava___

(10) ___Tricuspid Valve___

(11) ___Pulmonary Valve___

(12) ___(R) Pulmonary Veins___

(13) ___(R) Pulmonary Arteries___

(14) ___Superior Vena Cava___

Copyright ©2004, Elsevier. All rights reserved.

4. Cardiac cycle

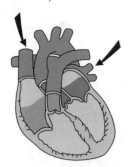

### 1. DIASTOLE
- Atria fill
- all valves closed

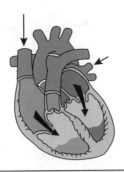

### 2. DIASTOLE
- increased arterial pressure opens AV valves
- ventricles fill

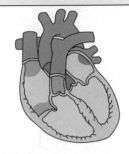

### 6. DIASTOLE
- ventricles empty
- ventricles relax
- aortic/pulmonary valves close

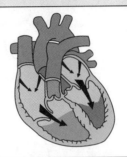

### 3. SYSTOLE BEGINS
- Atria contract/empty
- ventricles are full

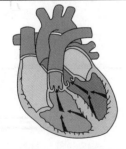

### 5. SYSTOLE
- ventricles contract
- ↑ pressure in ventricles
- aortic/pulmonary valves open
- blood ejected into aorta/ pulmonary artery

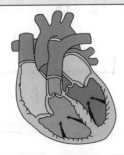

### 4. SYSTOLE
- ventricles begin contraction
- pressure closes AV valves
- atria relax

Copyright ©2004, Elsevier. All rights reserved.

5. Layers of the heart wall

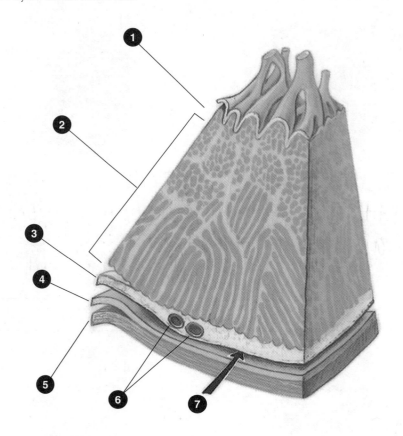

(1) Endocardium

(2) Myocardium

(3) Visceral pericardium (epicardium)

(4) Parietal pericardium

(5) Fibrous pericardium

(6) Coronary vessels

(7) Pericardial cavity

Copyright ©2004, Elsevier. All rights reserved.

6. Coronary arteries

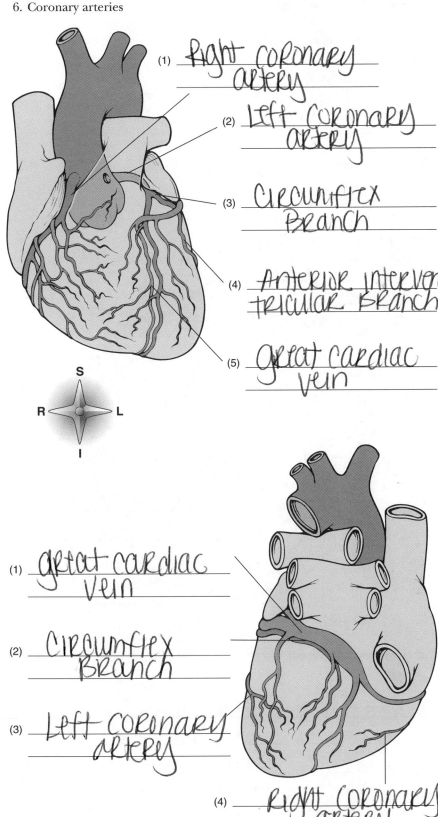

(1) Right coronary artery

(2) Left coronary artery

(3) Circumflex Branch

(4) Anterior interventricular Branch

(5) great cardiac vein

(1) great cardiac vein

(2) Circumflex Branch

(3) Left coronary artery

(4) Right coronary artery

Copyright ©2004, Elsevier. All rights reserved.

7. Conduction system of the heart

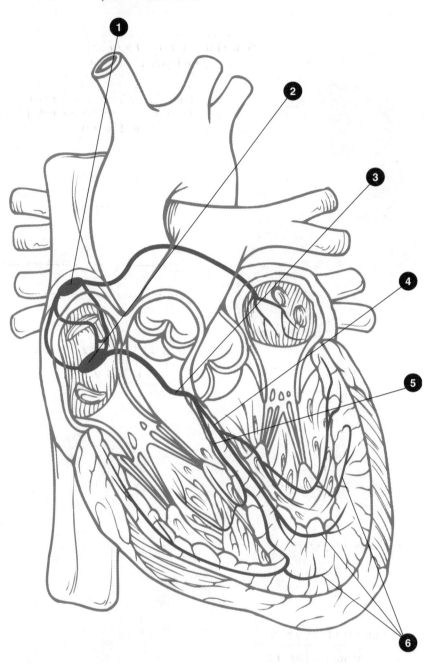

(1) Sinoatrial node

(2) Atrioventricular node

(3) Bundle of His

(4) Left Bundle Branch

(5) Right Bundle Branch

(6) Purkinje's fibers

Copyright ©2004, Elsevier. All rights reserved.

# PATIENT SCREENING

*For each scenario that follows, explain how and why you would schedule an appointment or suggest a referral based on the patient's reported symptoms.* ***First, review the "Guidelines for Patient-Screening Exercises" found on page iv in the "Introduction."***

1. A patient's wife calls in stating her husband just experienced the sudden onset of left-sided chest pain after exertion. The pain has radiated to the left arm. The pain was relieved when he stopped the strenuous activity and placed a nitroglycerin tablet under his tongue. She wants to know if the physician should see him. How do you handle this call?

_____

_____

_____

_____

_____

_____

2. A patient calls in saying she is experiencing headaches, lightheadedness, and dizziness. She took her blood pressure at an automatic blood pressure screening station at the pharmacy, and the reading was 168/98. How do you handle this phone call?

_____

_____

_____

_____

_____

_____

3. The husband of a patient calls in reporting his wife started having swollen feet and ankles, weight increase, and slight shortness of breath. She has a history of congestive heart failure. How do you handle this call?

_____

_____

_____

_____

_____

_____

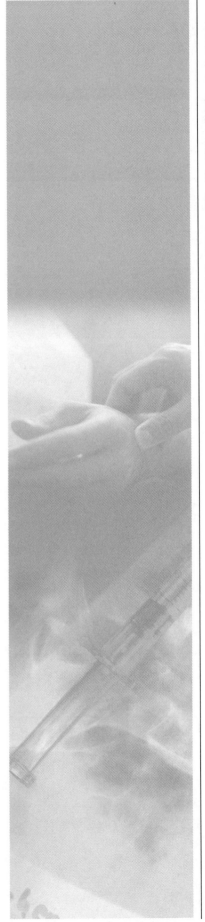

Copyright ©2004, Elsevier. All rights reserved.

4. The patient calls in reporting pain and tenderness in the left leg that is becoming more severe. She has noted swelling, redness, warmth, and the development of a tender cordlike mass under the skin. How do you handle this call?

_____

_____

_____

_____

_____

_____

5. The patient calls the office and says she is experiencing fatigue, and her skin—especially her hands—looks pale to her. She has had a few brief episodes of shortness of breath and a "pounding heart." How do you respond to this phone call?

_____

_____

_____

_____

_____

_____

_____

_____

# PATIENT TEACHING

*For each scenario below, outline the appropriate patient teaching you would perform.* ***First, review the "Guidelines for Patient-Teaching Exercises" found on page iv in the "Introduction."***

1. **CORONARY ARTERY DISEASE (CAD)**
   A patient has recently been diagnosed with CAD. She has returned to the office for additional patient teaching concerning this condition. The office has printed material outlining emergency medical intervention in the event of chest pain, as well as the prevention and control of the disorder. The physician requests you provide this material to the patient and review it with her. How do you approach this patient-teaching opportunity?

   _____

   _____

   _____

   _____

**124**

Copyright ©2004, Elsevier. All rights reserved.

## 2. HYPERTENSION

A patient diagnosed with hypertension is in the office for a blood pressure recheck. He makes the statement that because his blood pressure is much better today, it will be possible to stop taking the medication. The physician requests that you reinforce his instructions that the medication still needs to be taken on a regular basis. The office has printed material available to give to hypertensive patients. How do you approach this patient-teaching opportunity?

_____

_____

_____

_____

## 3. CONGESTIVE HEART FAILURE (CHF)

A patient is experiencing recurring CHF. The physician requests you reinforce his instructions to the patient and the family regarding treatment of the condition. How do you approach this patient-teaching opportunity?

_____

_____

_____

_____

## 4. ATHEROSCLEROSIS

A diagnosis of atherosclerosis has been confirmed. The physician requests your assistance in reinforcing her recommendations to the patient. The office has printed materials regarding this condition and you are instructed to review these with the patient. How do you approach this patient-teaching opportunity?

_____

_____

_____

_____

## 5. RAYNAUD PHENOMENON

It is a very cold day, and the patient has just seen the physician after a severe attack of her condition. Even though the physician has previously advised her about the importance of avoiding situations where she is exposed to severe cold, she continues to go outside without gloves and head covering. The physician requests you provide the patient with printed information concerning her condition and reinforce the fact that exposure to severe cold will cause severe pain. How do you approach this patient-teaching opportunity?

_____

_____

_____

_____

Copyright ©2004, Elsevier. All rights reserved.

# ESSAY QUESTION

*Write a response to the following question or statement. Use a separate sheet of paper if more space is needed.*

Describe the laboratory tests that are used to confirm a diagnosis of acute lymphocytic leukemia (ALL).

_____

_____

_____

_____

_____

_____

_____

_____

_____

_____

_____

_____

_____

_____

_____

_____

_____

_____

_____

_____

_____

_____

_____

_____

Copyright ©2004, Elsevier. All rights reserved.

# CERTIFICATION EXAMINATION REVIEW

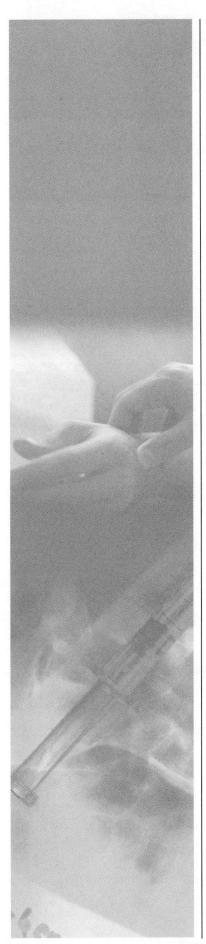

*Circle the letter of the choice that best completes the statement or answers the question.*

1. A person who complains of experiencing chest pain with exertion is having
   a. Angina pectoris
   b. A myocardial infarction
   c. Shortness of breath
   d. None of the above

2. Pericarditis is an inflammation of the
   a. Myocardium
   b. Endocardium
   c. Sac enclosing the heart
   d. None of the above

3. Raynaud phenomenon is a vasospastic disease that affects the
   a. Heart
   b. Legs and arms
   c. Hands, fingers, and feet
   d. None of the above

4. The diagnosis of anemia indicates that the patient is experiencing a reduction in
   a. Red blood cells or hemoglobin
   b. Platelets
   c. Lymphatic tissue
   d. None of the above

5. The hereditary blood disease, sickle cell anemia, is predominantly seen in
   a. The white race
   b. The black race
   c. Both a and b
   d. None of the above

6. The lymphatic tissue in Hodgkin's disease patients contains _____.
   a. Sickle cells
   b. Monocytes
   c. Reed-Sternberg cells
   d. None of the above

7. Rheumatic heart disease may cause problems with the
   a. Myocardium
   b. Valves
   c. Atria
   d. None of the above

8. Left-sided crushing chest pain, irregular heartbeat, dyspnea, and excessive sweating, nausea, anxiety, and denial are all symptoms of
   a. Mitral stenosis
   b. Angina pectoris
   c. Myocardial infarction
   d. All of the above

9. Electrocution, myocardial infarction, and drug overdose may cause
   a. Hypertension
   b. Cardiac arrest
   c. Cardiomyopathy
   d. None of the above

Copyright ©2004, Elsevier. All rights reserved.

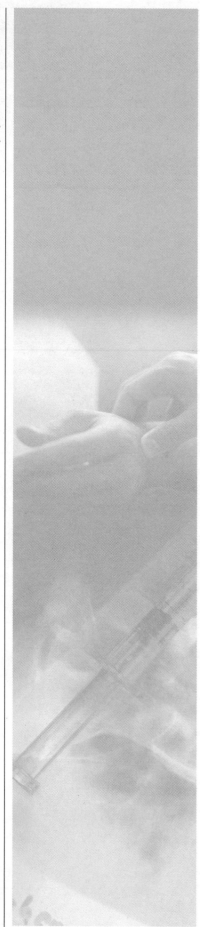

10. People with mitral valve prolapse are sometimes
    a. Asymptomatic
    b. Anxious
    c. Experiencing heart palpitations
    d. All of the above

11. Primary or essential hypertension
    a. Is related to lifestyle habits
    b. Is genetic
    c. Has an unknown cause
    d. None of the above

12. Ischemia causes
    a. Death to tissue
    b. Swelling of tissue
    c. Blood disorders
    d. None of the above

13. Blood transfusion incompatibility reactions are
    a. Potentially life threatening
    b. Always fatal
    c. A common problem
    d. None of the above

14. Lymphedema causes swelling of
    a. The heart
    b. An extremity
    c. Heart valves
    d. None of the above

15. Cardiac arrhythmias are the result of
    a. Smoking
    b. Fat deposits
    c. Interference with the conduction system of the heart
    d. None of the above

Copyright ©2004, Elsevier. All rights reserved.

# CHAPTER 11

# Diseases and Conditions of the Urinary System

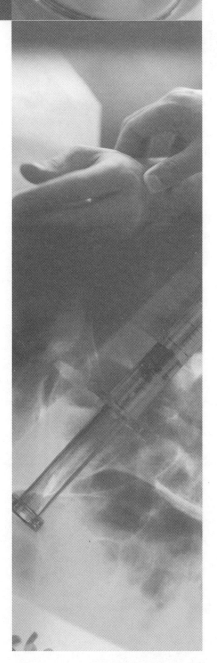

## WORD DEFINITIONS

*Define the following basic medical terms:*

1. ARF _____

2. Anorexia _____

3. BUN _____

4. Calculi _____

5. Casts _____

6. Extracellular _____

7. Flank _____

8. Intrarenal _____

9. IVP _____

10. Lethargic _____

11. Nephrolithotomy _____

12. Neuropathies _____

13. Oliguria _____

14. Pitting edema _____

15. Proteinuria _____

16. Renin _____

17. Spontaneously _____

18. Urgency _____

Copyright ©2004, Elsevier. All rights reserved.

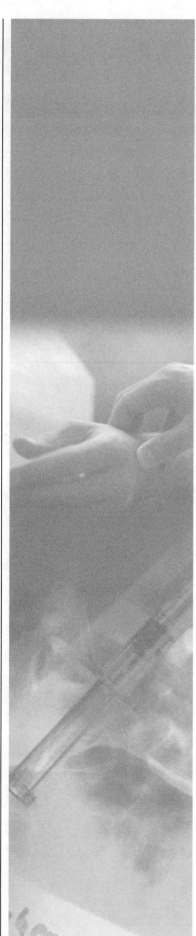

# GLOSSARY TERMS

*Define the following chapter glossary terms:*

1. Azotemia — excess of urea or other nitrogenous bodies in the blood

2. BUN — measurement of urea nitrogen in the serum or plasma

3. Calculi — stone usually composed of mineral salts / calcified de on the feet

4. Clean-catch urine specimen — urine specimen obtained by cleaning the genitalia & then capturing a midstream urine sample 4 lab.

5. Dialysis — procedure that filters out unwanted substances from the blood, usually in cases of Renal fail

6. Erythrocyte sedimentation rate (ESR) — measurable Reflection of the acute-phase Reaction in inflammation & infection

7. Fibrotic — abnormal formation of fibrous tissue

8. Glomerulosclerosis — hardening of the Renal glomerulus

9. Glomeruli — tiny ball of microscopic blood vessels on the end of the Renal tubules

10. Hematuria — blood in the urine

11. Hypoalbuminemia — low albumin levels in the blood

12. Idiopathic — Refers to a disease w/o a known cause

13. Intravenous pyelograms — Radiographic study of the Renal pelvis & u. Reter using injected dye

14. Intravenous urogram — Radiographic study of the urinary tract using injected dye

15. Malaise — feeling of discomfort, illness or uneasiness

16. Metabolic acidosis — excessive acid in the body fluids caused by dehydration etc.

17. Nephrons — functioning unit of the Kidney / Renal tubule

18. Pyelonephritis — purulent infection of the Kidney tissue and Renal pelvis

19. Renal calculi — Kidney stones

20. Uremia — toxic condition of excessive waste product protein, nitrogen in the blood caused by Renal insufficiency

Copyright ©2004, Elsevier. All rights reserved.

# SHORT ANSWER

*Answer the following questions:*

1. Can chronic glomerulonephritis lead to renal failure?

   _____

2. What diagnostic test is often ordered to evaluate the function of the urinary system?

   _____

3. What usually precedes acute glomerulonephritis?

   _____

4. Name the procedure used to examine the urinary tract.

   _____

5. Regardless of the size of the stone, are symptoms of renal calculi the same?

   _____

6. What is the most common type of kidney disease?

   _____

7. List causes of neurogenic bladder.

   _____

8. Describe hematuria.

   _____

9. List the functions of the urinary system.

   _____

10. Pressure from urine that cannot flow past an obstruction in the urinary tract causes what condition affecting the kidney?

    _____

11. List types of nephrotoxic agents that commonly cause renal damage.

    _____

    _____

12. Name the treatment of choice for renal cell carcinoma.

    _____

13. Define nephrotic syndrome.

    _____

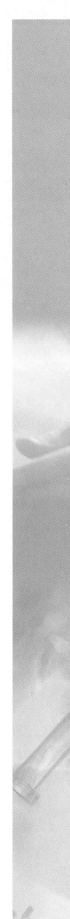

Copyright ©2004, Elsevier. All rights reserved.

14. Glomerulosclerosis results from what disease?

_____

15. List usual causes of cystitis and urethritis.

_____

_____

16. In relation to the urinary system, list the occasions when catheterization may be indicated.

_____

_____

17. Define pyuria.

_____

18. List the symptoms of acute glomerulonephritis.

_____

19. List factors that may lead to stress incontinence (enuresis).

_____

_____

20. Identify the cause of bladder cancer.

_____

21. Describe the sequence of events when a patient has acute renal failure.

_____

_____

22. After what length of time will a kidney fail to function if an obstruction is not resolved when the patient has hydronephrosis?

_____

23. Explain the usual treatment of renal calculi.

_____

24. Identify the cause of polycystic kidney disease.

_____

25. Describe the appearance of a polycystic kidney.

_____

_____

Copyright ©2004, Elsevier. All rights reserved.

# FILL IN THE BLANKS

*Fill in the blanks with the correct terms. A Word List has been provided. Words used twice are indicated with a (2).*

1. With renal cell carcinoma, the malignancy can begin in the _____ or be secondary to carcinoma elsewhere in the body.

2. The urinary system is responsible for __producing__, __storing__, and __exceeting__ __urine__.

3. The functional unit of the kidney is the _____.

4. The three functional processes of the kidney in the manufacture of urine are _____, _____, and _____.

5. Urine is stored in the _____.

6. Function of the urinary system is evaluated by __urinalysis__ and __blood__ __tests__.

7. Four symptoms of urinary disease are __nausea__, __bloody__ __urine__, _____ _____, and __hypertension__.

8. _____ _____ is an inflammation and swelling of the glomeruli.

9. The major structures of the urinary system consist of __oliguria__ _____, two _____, the _____ _____, and the _____.

10. Nephrotic syndrome encompasses a group of symptoms referred to as _____ _____ kidney.

11. Initial symptoms of acute renal failure include __oliguria__, __gastrointestinal disturbances__, __headache__, __drowsiness__, and other alterations in the level of consciousness.

12. The treatment of choice for pyelonephritis consists of intravenous or oral __antibiotics__, usually __penicillin__ or __cephalosporin__, given for a full 7 to __10__ days.

Copyright ©2004, Elsevier. All rights reserved.

13. Kidney stones form when there is an excessive amount of

    _Calcium_ or _uric acid_ in the blood.

14. Diabetic patients vary in their susceptibility to renal

    _____, so the treatment plan for diabetic glomeru-

    losclerosis is _____ for each person.

15. The treatment for neurogenic bladder is directed toward prevention of

    _____ and attempts to restore some _____

    in function.

## WORD LIST

~~10,~~ acute glomerulonephritis, ~~antibiotics,~~ bladder, ~~blood tests,~~ ~~bloody urine,~~ ~~calcium,~~ ~~cephalosporin,~~ decreased urinary output, ~~drowsiness,~~ excreting urine, failure, filtration, ~~gastrointestinal disturbances,~~ ~~headache,~~ ~~hypertension,~~ individualized, kidneys (2), ~~nausea,~~ nephron, normalcy, ~~oliguria,~~ ~~penicillin,~~ ~~producing,~~ protein losing, reabsorption, secretion, ~~storing,~~ ureters, urethra, ~~uric acid,~~ ~~urinalysis,~~ urinary bladder, urinary tract infections (UTIs)

## ANATOMIC STRUCTURES

*Identify the structures in the following anatomic diagrams. For number 4, identify the three phases of urine formation.*

1. The urinary system

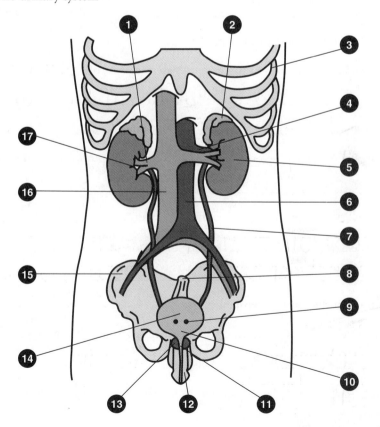

Copyright ©2004, Elsevier. All rights reserved.

(1) Renal vein  
(2) adrenal gland  
(3) Ribs  
(4) Renal artery  
(5) kidney (left)  
(6) Aorta  
(7) Ureter  
(8) Rectum  
(9) Ureteral Opening  

(10) Trigone  
(11) Urethra  
(12) Penis  
(13) Prostate gland  
(14) Urinary Bladder  
(15) Pelvis  
(16) Inferior Vena Cava  
(17) Hilum  

2. Internal structure of the kidney

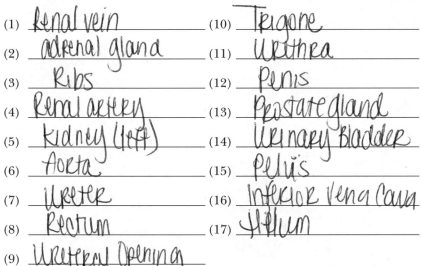
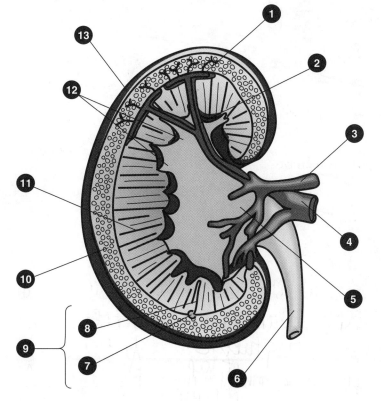

(1) Arcuate Artery  
(2) Interlobar artery  
(3) Renal Artery  
(4) Renal Vein  
(5) Renal pelvis  
(6) Ureter  
(7) glomerulus  

(8) Tubule  
(9) Nephron  
(10) Renal Cortex  
(11) Renal Medulla  
(12) Calyx  
(13) Renal Capsule  

Copyright ©2004, Elsevier. All rights reserved.

3. The nephron

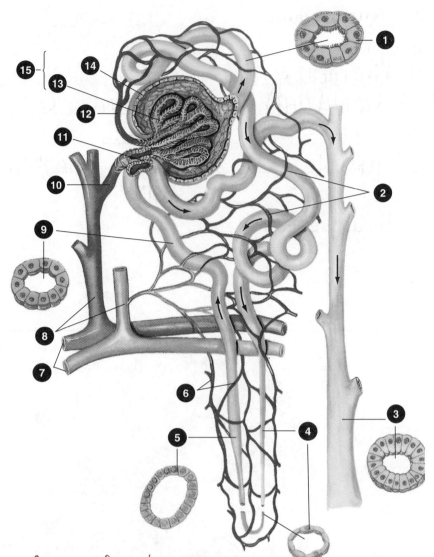

(1) Proximal Convoluted Tubule (9) Distal Convoluted tubule

(2) Peritubular Capillaries (10) Afferent Arteriole

(3) Collecting tubule (11) Juxtaglomerular Apparatus

(4) Descending limb of loop of Henle (12) Efferent Arteriole

(5) Ascending limb of loop of Henle (13) Glomerulus

(6) Peritubular Capillaries (14) Bowman's Capsule

(7) Arcuate Artery & Vein (15) Renal Corpuscle

(8) Interlobular Artery & Vein

Copyright ©2004, Elsevier. All rights reserved.

4. Formation of urine

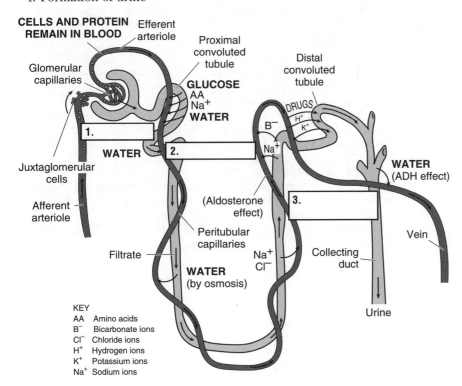

**CELLS AND PROTEIN REMAIN IN BLOOD**

Efferent arteriole

Glomerular capillaries

Proximal convoluted tubule

**GLUCOSE**
AA
Na⁺
**WATER**

Distal convoluted tubule

DRUGS
H⁺
K⁺

B⁻

Na⁺

1.

**WATER**

2.

Juxtaglomerular cells

Afferent arteriole

(Aldosterone effect)

3.

**WATER** (ADH effect)

Vein

Peritubular capillaries

Filtrate

Na⁺
Cl⁻

Collecting duct

**WATER** (by osmosis)

Urine

KEY
AA   Amino acids
B⁻   Bicarbonate ions
Cl⁻  Chloride ions
H⁺   Hydrogen ions
K⁺   Potassium ions
Na⁺  Sodium ions

# PATIENT SCREENING

*For each scenario below, explain how and why you would schedule an appointment or suggest a referral based on the patient's reported symptoms. **First, review the "Guidelines for Patient-Screening Exercises" found on page iv in the "Introduction."***

1. A mother calls in reporting her daughter has experienced a sudden onset of grossly bloody urine. The urine is dark and is described as being coffee-colored. The child had a streptococcal infection 1 to 2 weeks ago. The child also is complaining of a headache, has a loss of appetite, and a low-grade fever. Flank or back pain is an additional complaint of the child. How do you handle this call?

   _____

   _____

   _____

   _____

2. A patient reports she has experienced rapid onset of fever, chills, nausea and vomiting, and flank (lumbar) pain. She had a UTI with urinary frequency and urgency last week. The patient reports a foul odor to the urine with possible blood and pus. There is tenderness in the suprapubic region. How do you handle this call?

   _____

   _____

   _____

   _____

Copyright ©2004, Elsevier. All rights reserved.

3. A patient calls in advising he has experienced sudden severe pain in the flank area and urinary urgency. He also is complaining of nausea and vomiting, blood in the urine, fever, chills, and abdominal distention. How do you respond to this phone call?

_____

_____

_____

_____

4. A female patient calls the office complaining of urinary urgency, frequency, and even incontinence. Additionally, she says she has pain in the pelvic region and low back, spasm of the bladder, fever and chills, and a burning sensation with urination. Her urine is dark yellow. How do you respond to this phone call?

_____

_____

_____

_____

5. A female patient advises she is experiencing leakage of urine on coughing, sneezing, laughing, lifting, or running, without prior urgency. The patient is unable to control the leakage during physical exertion. How do you handle this call?

_____

_____

_____

_____

## PATIENT TEACHING

*For each scenario below, outline the appropriate patient teaching you would perform. First, review the "Guidelines for Patient-Teaching Exercises" found on page iv in the "Introduction."*

1. **ACUTE GLOMERULONEPHRITIS**
   A patient has recently been diagnosed with acute glomerulonephritis. Antibiotics have been prescribed. The physician has printed instructions for patients with this condition. You are asked to provide the patient and family with the printed information and review it with them. How do you approach this patient-teaching opportunity?

_____

_____

_____

_____

Copyright ©2004, Elsevier. All rights reserved.

2. **PYELONEPHRITIS**

A female patient has a recurring occurrence of pyelonephritis. The physician has requested you to provide and review this material with the patient. How do you approach this patient-teaching opportunity?

_____

_____

_____

_____

3. **RENAL CALCULI**

A patient complains of sudden onset of severe flank pain accompanied by pelvic pressure. Radiographs indicate the presence of renal calculi. The physician requests you to provide the patient with printed information concerning renal calculi therapy. How do you approach this patient-teaching opportunity?

_____

_____

_____

_____

4. **DIABETIC NEPHROPATHY**

A patient has recently been diagnosed with diabetic neuropathy. He is somewhat confused about this complication of his diabetes. The physician has written information for this type of disorder. You are instructed to provide him with the printed information and to review its contents with him. How do you approach this patient-teaching opportunity?

_____

_____

_____

_____

5. **STRESS INCONTINENCE**

A female patient has been experiencing stress incontinence. The physician has printed instructions to help patients deal with this condition. The physician requests that you provide the instructions to the patient and that you review them with her. How do you approach this patient-teaching opportunity?

_____

_____

_____

_____

Copyright ©2004, Elsevier. All rights reserved.

# ESSAY QUESTION

*Write a response to the following question or statement. Use a separate sheet of paper if more space is needed.*

Compare hemodialysis and peritoneal dialysis.

_____

_____

_____

_____

_____

_____

_____

_____

_____

_____

_____

_____

_____

_____

_____

_____

_____

_____

_____

_____

_____

_____

_____

_____

_____

Copyright ©2004, Elsevier. All rights reserved.

# CERTIFICATION EXAMINATION REVIEW

*Circle the letter of the choice that best completes the statement or answers the question.*

1. Obstructive diseases of the kidney may be caused by
   a. Metabolic disorders
   b. Congenital or structural defects
   c. Immunologic disorders
   d. None of the above

2. The most common type of renal disease is
   a. Acute renal failure
   b. Nephrosis
   c. Pyelonephritis
   d. Hydronephrosis

3. Symptoms of cystitis include
   a. Urinary urgency, frequency, and incontinence
   b. Pelvic pain
   c. Burning with urination
   d. All of the above

4. Group A beta hemolytic streptococcus may precede
   a. Hydronephrosis
   b. Acute renal failure
   c. Acute glomerulonephritis
   d. None of the above

5. Lithotripsy, relief of pain, surgical intervention, increased fluid intake, and diuretics are all ways of treating
   a. Hydronephrosis
   b. Renal calculi
   c. Glomerulonephritis
   d. All of the above

6. An ascending bacterial invasion of the urinary tract can cause
   a. Renal calculi
   b. Hydronephrosis
   c. Cystitis and urethritis
   d. All of the above

7. Chronic glomerulonephritis is
   a. Slowly progressive and infectious
   b. Slowly progressive and noninfectious
   c. Not progressive
   d. None of the above

8. Enuresis is caused from a weakening of the
   a. Pelvic floor muscles
   b. Urethral structure
   c. Both a and b
   d. None of the above

9. Solvents, heavy metals, antibiotics, pesticides, and mushrooms are known to
   a. Cause renal damage
   b. Cause cystitis
   c. Cause pyelonephritis
   d. None of the above

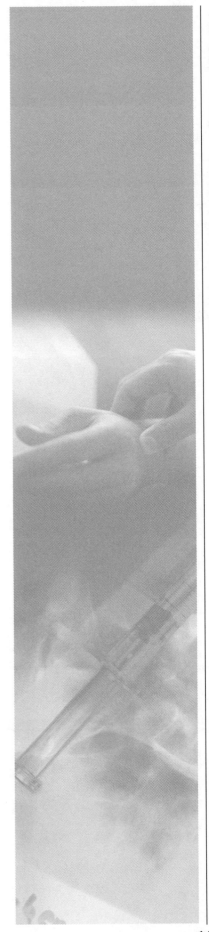

Copyright ©2004, Elsevier. All rights reserved.

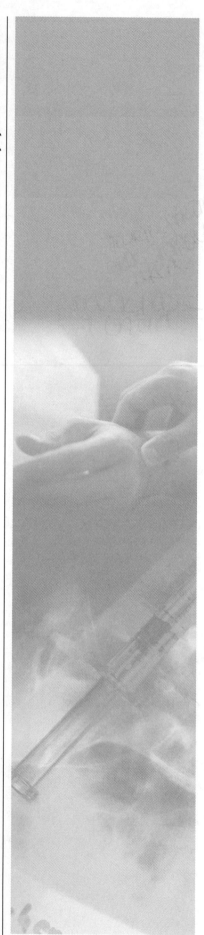

10. Smoking, obesity, and prolonged exposure to chemicals such as asbestos and cadmium are risk factors associated with
    a. Polycystic kidney disease
    b. Renal cell carcinoma
    c. Glomerulonephritis
    d. None of the above

11. Pus in the urine is called
    a. Azotemia
    b. Pyuria
    c. Cystitis
    d. None of the above

12. Hematuria is
    a. Bacteria in the urine
    b. Blood in the urine
    c. Fat in the urine
    d. None of the above

13. Azotemia is
    a. A drug that promotes urine output
    b. Excess urea in the blood ·
    c. Excess urea in the urine
    d. None of the above

14. A clinical emergency that involves the renal system is
    a. Cystitis
    b. Hematuria
    c. Acute renal failure
    d. Pyuria

Copyright ©2004, Elsevier. All rights reserved.

**CHAPTER 12**

# Diseases and Conditions of the Reproductive System

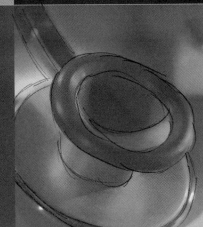

## WORD DEFINITIONS

*Define the following basic medical terms:*

1. Amenorrhea — *absence of your period*

2. Anomaly — *deviation from normal esp. if a bodily part*

3. Axillary — *located near the axilla*

4. Cervicitis — *inflam. of the uterine cervix*

5. Cystitis — *inflam. of the urinary bladder*

6. Cystoscopy — *use of the cystoscope to examine the bladder*

7. Degenerative — *involving degeneration of the nervous system*

8. Endometrial — *consisting of a endometrium*

9. Lymphectomy — *to take out the lymph*

10. Melena —

11. Nocturia — *urination @ night*

12. Noninvasive — *not tending to spread*

13. Proctoscopy — *dialation / visual inspection of the rectum*

14. Prostatitis — *inflamation of the prostate gland*

15. Septicemia — *bacteria in the blood*

16. Urethritis — *inflamation of the urethra*

Copyright ©2004, Elsevier. All rights reserved.

# GLOSSARY TERMS

*Define the following chapter glossary terms:*

1. Abruptio placentae — detatchment of the placenta from ~~uterus~~ *before birth*
2. Amniotic fluid — transparent albuminous liquid made by the amnion ~~the fetus~~
3. Asymptomatic — w/o symptoms
4. Colporrhaphy — suturing of the vagina
5. Endometrium — lining of the uterus
6. Laparoscopy — surgical procedure to examine the abdomen using indoscope *looking from the stomach area*
7. Neoplasm — abnormal formation of new tissue
8. Nulliparous — woman who has never produced viable offspring *never has a child*
9. Pathologist — Dr. who specializes in the study of disease
10. Peau d'orange — condition where skin is dimpled
11. Pelvic inflammatory disease — inflamation of the female pelvic organ
12. Peritonitis — inflamation of the membrane that lines the abdominal cavity
13. Prostate-specific antigen (PSA) — enzyme that is measured in a blood test to detect prostate cancer
14. Serologic — study of blood serum to measure antibodies
15. Zygote — fertilized ovum

# SHORT ANSWER

*Answer the following questions:*

1. Name the male reproductive organs that produce sperm.

2. Identify the drug of choice to treat syphilis.

3. List the signs and symptoms of preeclampsia in pregnancy.

4. Identify first sign of testicular cancer.

Copyright ©2004, Elsevier. All rights reserved.

5. What is dysmenorrhea?

   _____

6. Name the term for pain that occurs at ovulation.

   _____

7. Name the sexually transmitted disease that is referred to as the "silent STD."

   _____

8. Identify the treatment for condylomata.

   _____

9. What happens during placenta previa?

   _____

10. Identify the second leading cause of cancer deaths among women.

    _____

11. What is the best prevention of epididymitis?

    _____

12. Identify the treatment for testicular torsion.

    _____

13. List complications of benign prostatic hypertrophy.

    _____

14. Testicular cancer is most common in men of what age?

    _____

15. Cite causes of secondary dysmenorrhea.

    _____

16. What is a leiomyoma?

    _____

17. What is included in the initial diagnostic evaluation for prostatic cancer?

    _____

    _____

18. Is dyspareunia more common in men or women?

    _____

19. Identify the main goals of treatment for genital herpes.

    _____

Copyright ©2004, Elsevier. All rights reserved.

20. By what route is herpes transmitted?

_____

21. Are physical problems always the cause of impotence?

_____

22. With regular unprotected intercourse for 1 year, what percentage of couples is able to conceive?

_____

23. What is the age range in which most women are diagnosed with ovarian cancer?

_____

24. Identify the time during pregnancy that most women experience morning sickness.

_____

25. With ectopic pregnancy, where does the fertilized ovum usually implant?

_____

26. List the characteristics of eclampsia.

_____

27. Is there usually a fetus present with a hydatidiform mole?

_____

28. Is cystic disease of the breast benign or cancerous?

_____

# FILL IN THE BLANKS

*Fill in the blanks with the correct terms. A Word List has been provided.*

1. Sperm is transported from the testes through the series of ducts beginning with the epididymis, the _____ _____, and the _____ ducts.

2. The _____ are accessory organs of _____ and are two milk-producing glands.

3. Sexually transmitted disease (STD) rates in the _____ _____ are among the highest in the world and are growing.

Copyright ©2004, Elsevier. All rights reserved.

4. Trichomoniasis is a _____ infection of the

   _____ genitourinary tract.

5. Genital warts are usually painless, but they may _____

   or _____ .

6. The most common diseases of the male reproductive system are those

   affecting the _____ gland.

7. _____ or _____ infection or

   _____ causes inflammation of the testes.

8. Endometriosis is considered a benign condition but the severe symptoms

   are _____ and _____ .

9. Leiomyomas and _____ are the most common

   _____ of the female reproductive system.

10. Toxic shock syndrome is an _____, _____

    infection with exotoxin producing _____ of

    *Staphylococcus aureus.*

11. Many _____ experience the onset of menopause

    between the ages of _____ and _____ .

12. Prolapse of the uterus is a _____ displacement of the

    _____ from its normal location in the body.

13. A _____ is a downward displacement of the urinary

    bladder into the _____ wall of the vagina.

14. Exercises to strengthen the pelvic floor muscles are called

    _____ exercises.

15. Mastitis is frequently caused by a _____ or

    _____ infection.

## WORD LIST

45, 55, acute, anterior, bacterial, breast, burn, chronic, cystocele, downward, ductus deferens, ejaculatory, fibroids, injury, itch, Kegel, lower, painful, prostate, protozoal, reproduction, staphylococcal, strains, streptococcal, systemic, tumors, United States, uterus, viral, women

Copyright ©2004, Elsevier. All rights reserved.

# ANATOMIC STRUCTURES

*Identify the structures in the following anatomic diagrams.*

1. Normal male reproductive system

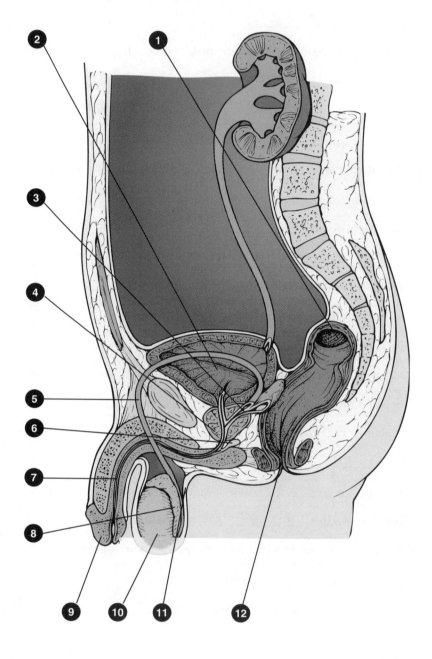

(1) _____    (7) _____

(2) _____    (8) _____

(3) _____    (9) _____

(4) _____    (10) _____

(5) _____    (11) _____

(6) _____    (12) _____

Copyright ©2004, Elsevier. All rights reserved.

2. Normal female reproductive system

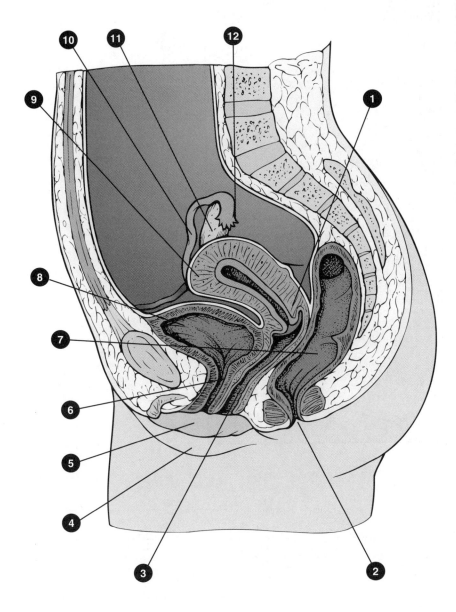

(1) _____     (7) _____

(2) _____     (8) _____

(3) _____     (9) _____

(4) _____     (10) _____

(5) _____     (11) _____

(6) _____     (12) _____

Copyright ©2004, Elsevier. All rights reserved.

3. Normal female breast

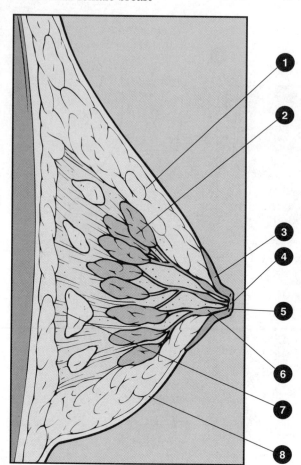

(1) _____

(2) _____

(3) _____

(4) _____

(5) _____

(6) _____

(7) _____

(8) _____

Copyright ©2004, Elsevier. All rights reserved.

# PATIENT SCREENING

*For each scenario below, explain how and why you would schedule an appointment or suggest a referral based on the patient's reported symptoms.* **First, review the "Guidelines for Patient-Screening Exercises" found on page iv in the "Introduction."**

1. A female patient calls in requesting an appointment saying she is experiencing painful urination and severe itching in the perineal region. How do you respond to her call?

   _____

   _____

   _____

2. A 60-year-old male patient calls the office advising he is experiencing urinary frequency including nocturia. How do you handle this call?

   _____

   _____

   _____

3. A female patient calls advising she is experiencing fever, chills, a foul-smelling vaginal discharge, backache, and a painful, tender abdomen. How do you handle this call?

   _____

   _____

   _____

4. A female patient's husband calls the office saying his wife is 2 months pregnant and has developed vaginal bleeding and cramping pelvic pain. How do you handle this call?

   _____

   _____

   _____

5. A female patient calls in requesting an appointment stating she has been experiencing an uncomfortable feeling in her breasts. She found a lump this morning in her right breast. How do you handle this call?

   _____

   _____

   _____

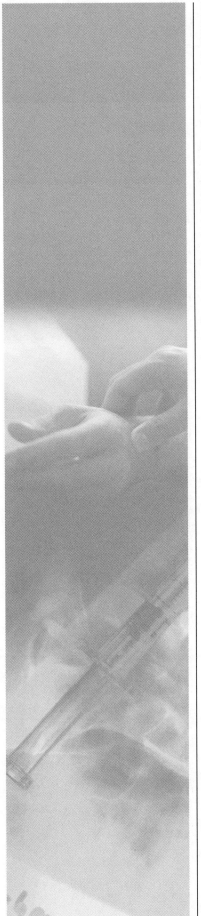

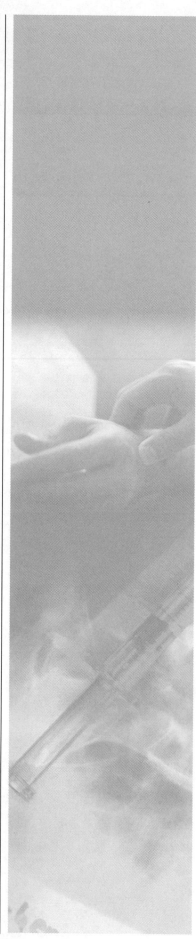

# PATIENT TEACHING

*For each scenario below, outline the appropriate patient teaching you would perform.*
***First, review the "Guidelines for Patient-Teaching Exercises" found on page iv in the***
***"Introduction."***

1. **SYPHILIS**

   A patient has been diagnosed with syphilis. The practice has printed
   instructions for patients diagnosed with this condition. The physician has
   instructed you to provide the patient with the printed information and to
   review it with her. How do you approach this patient-teaching opportunity?

   _____

   _____

   _____

   _____

   _____

   _____

2. **ORCHITIS**

   A young male patient has just been diagnosed with orchitis. The physician requests you provide the patient with the printed information concerning this condition. How do you approach this patient-teaching
   opportunity?

   _____

   _____

   _____

   _____

   _____

   _____

3. **PREMENSTRUAL SYNDROME (PMS)**

   A female patient complains of typical premenstrual syndrome symptoms.
   The office has printed information for patient teaching about this condition. The physician requests you to provide the information sheets to the
   patient and review them with her. How do you approach this patient-
   teaching opportunity?

   _____

   _____

   _____

   _____

   _____

   _____

Copyright ©2004, Elsevier. All rights reserved.

4. **ENDOMETRIOSIS**

   A young female patient has been complaining of intolerable menstrual cramps and other pelvic pain. The diagnosis of endometriosis has been made. The physician has written instructions for this condition. You are instructed to provide the patient with the printed material and review it with her. How do you approach this patient-teaching opportunity?

   _____

   _____

   _____

   _____

   _____

   _____

5. **PREECLAMPSIA (TOXEMIA)**

   A pregnant patient has been experiencing elevated blood pressure and sudden weight gain. She has been diagnosed with preeclampsia. The physician has printed instructions for this condition. You are instructed to provide this information to the patient and her family. How do you approach this patient-teaching opportunity?

   _____

   _____

   _____

   _____

   _____

   _____

Copyright ©2004, Elsevier. All rights reserved.

# ESSAY QUESTION

*Write a response to the following question or statement. Use a separate sheet of paper if more space is needed.*

Discuss the cause, symptoms and signs, and treatment of premature labor.

_____

_____

_____

_____

_____

_____

_____

_____

_____

_____

_____

_____

_____

_____

_____

_____

_____

_____

_____

_____

_____

_____

# CERTIFICATION EXAMINATION REVIEW

*Circle the letter of the choice that best completes the statement or answers the question.*

1. Genital warts and many different types of cancer develop from
   a. Syphilis
   b. HPV
   c. Chlamydia
   d. None of the above

Copyright ©2004, Elsevier. All rights reserved.

2. Pelvic inflammatory disease, septicemia, and septic arthritis are complications that may develop from untreated
   a. Syphilis
   b. Human papilloma virus (HPV)
   c. Gonorrhea
   d. None of the above

3. When functioning endometrial tissue is present outside the uterine cavity, the condition is called _____.
   a. Septicemia
   b. Gonorrhea
   c. Uterine cancer
   d. None of the above

4. Dyspareunia is more common in
   a. Men
   b. Women
   c. Teenagers
   d. Toddlers

5. Impotence may be caused from
   a. Use of recreational drugs
   b. Use of hypertensive medications
   c. Drinking alcohol
   d. All of the above

6. Protrusion of the rectum into the bladder is a
   a. Cystocele
   b. Rectal fissure
   c. Rectocele
   d. None of the above

7. Pain that occurs at ovulation is called
   a. Premenstrual syndrome
   b. Mittelschmerz
   c. Both a and b
   d. None of the above

8. A Pap smear may be a valuable tool in diagnosing
   a. Cervical cancer
   b. Breast cancer
   c. Testicular cancer
   d. All of the above

9. Herpes simplex virus
   a. Is not curable
   b. Is easily treated
   c. Is only detected by a Pap smear
   d. None of the above

10. A digital rectal examination, blood test for prostate-specific antigen (PSA), and a biopsy to confirm are all evaluations for
   a. Prostate cancer
   b. Testicular cancer
   c. Bladder cancer
   d. None of the above

Copyright ©2004, Elsevier. All rights reserved.

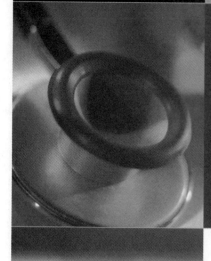

# CHAPTER 13

# Neurologic Diseases and Conditions

## WORD DEFINITIONS

*Define the following basic medical terms:*

1. Bradycardia — slow ♥ rate.

2. Cephalgia — headache

3. Craniotomy — surgical opening of the skull to enlarge.

4. Dilated —

5. Dysarthric — difficulty in articulating words due 2 disease of the CNS (central nerv system

6. Empyema — presence of pus in a bodily cavity

7. Flaccid — not firm/stiff

8. Hemicranial — pain in 1 side of the head

9. Hemiparesis — muscular weakness

10. Hypotension — low bp

11. Intervertebral — situated between vertebrae

12. Intracranial — situated w/in the cranium

13. Laminectomy — surgical removal of the posterior arch of a vertebra

14. Photophobia — tolerence to light

15. Sequela — aftereffect of disease/treatment

16. Syncope — loss of consciousness resulting from insufficient blood flood to the brain

Copyright ©2004, Elsevier. All rights reserved.

# GLOSSARY TERMS

*Define the following chapter glossary terms:*

1. Autosomal — any of the 22 ordinary paired chromosome in humans

2. Cauterize — 

3. Demyelination — loss of the myelin sheath of a nerve

4. Diplopia — double vision

5. Encephalitis — inflammation of the brain

6. Ergot — drug obtained from a fungus that grows on rye plants

7. Fibrin — protein material produced by the action of thrombin on fibrinogen

8. Foramen — opening/hole in bone allowing the passage of nerves/blood vessels

9. Hemiparesis — paralysis affecting 1 side of the body

10. Intractable — incurable/resistant to treatment

11. Lumbar puncture — surgical procedure to w/draw spinal fluid for analysis

12. Neurotransmitter — chemical released by the terminal end fibers of an axon

13. Nuchal rigidity — neck stiffness

14. Paresis — partial paralysis

15. Plasmapheresis — process of separating blood into its components by centrifuging

# SHORT ANSWER

*Answer the following questions:*

1. Identify the difference between efferent and afferent nerves.

_____

_____

2. Identify the cause of cerebrovascular accidents.

_____

_____

3. Cite another name for a transient ischemic attack (TIA).

_____

4. Does a TIA usually cause unconsciousness?

_____

Copyright ©2004, Elsevier. All rights reserved.

5. Which is more serious, a concussion or a cerebral contusion?

_____

6. Identify the common complication of a depressed skull fracture.

_____

_____

7. Identify the most frequent cause of a depressed skull.

_____

_____

8. What is the goal of treatment for spinal cord injuries?

_____

_____

9. List the symptoms of degenerative disk disease.

_____

_____

_____

10. Name the function of an intervertebral disk.

_____

11. Is sciatic nerve injury considered a pathological condition?

_____

12. If a person is having seizures, does it always mean they have epilepsy?

_____

13. Identify the type of medications that are used to treat epilepsy.

_____

14. Encephalitis is usually the result of a bite from what insect?

_____

15. List possible treatments for a brain abscess.

_____

16. Explain why a lumbar puncture is contraindicated if the patient has a brain abscess.

_____

Copyright ©2004, Elsevier. All rights reserved.

17. Identify the symptoms of Guillain-Barre syndrome.

_____

_____

18. Identify the vaccines that have helped eliminate cases of poliomyelitis.

_____

19. Cite the statistics for overall 5-year survival of all types of brain tumors.

_____

20. Identify the area of the skull involved with a basilar skull fracture.

_____

21. What physical manifestations alert the physician to order images of the cranial vault to investigate for a basilar skull fracture?

_____

22. Name the possible routes through which the poliomyelitis virus may enter the body.

_____

23. How are primary brain tumors classified?

_____

24. Identify the race having the highest incidence of brain tumors.

_____

25. How are the cranial nerves assessed during a neurologic examination?

_____

_____

_____

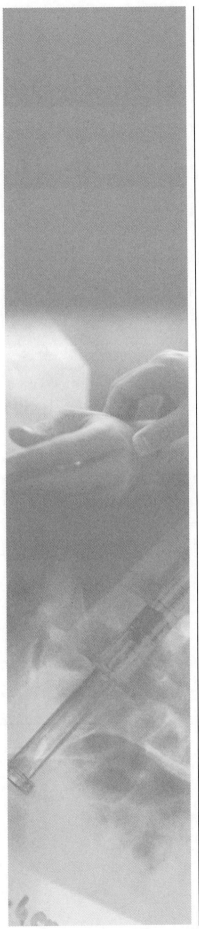

Copyright ©2004, Elsevier. All rights reserved.

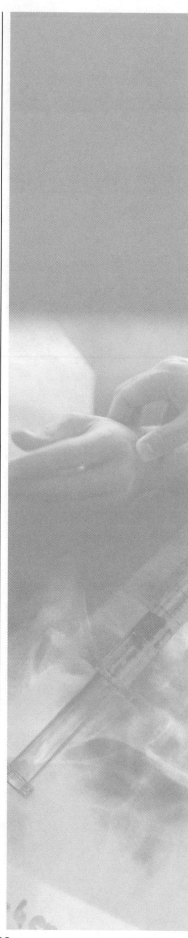

# FILL IN THE BLANKS

*Fill in the blanks with the correct terms. A Word List has been provided. Words used twice are indicated with a (2).*

1. Electrical impulses are carried throughout the body by ___neurons___.

2. The two divisions of the nervous system are the ___central___ nervous system and the ___peripheral___ nervous system.

3. The central nervous system (CNS) includes the ___brain___ and ___spinal cord___.

4. Five pairs of the ___12___ cranial nerves originate in the ___medulla oblongata___, an extension of the spinal cord.

5. The ___spinal cord___ is divided into 31 segments.

6. A cerebral concussion is a _____ of the cerebral tissue that is caused by _____ back and forth movement of the head as in an acceleration-deceleration insult.

7. A contusion of the brain is caused by a _____ to the _____ or an _____ against a hard surface, as in an automobile accident.

8. When a portion of the skull is broken and pushed in on the brain causing injury, it is said to be a _____ skull fracture.

9. Quadriplegia results in paralysis of the _____ _____ and usually the trunk.

10. Intervertebral disks are soft pads of _____ located between each vertebrae that make up the _____.

11. Headaches may be acute or chronic and located in the _____, _____, or _____ regions of the head.

12. Before the onset of a headache, many persons who experience _____ headaches have visual auras.

Copyright ©2004, Elsevier. All rights reserved.

13. Partial seizures do not involve the _____ brain but

    arise from a _____ area in the brain.

14. Anticonvulsant medications are the treatment of choice for

    _____.

15. Patients with amyotrophic lateral sclerosis (ALS) have difficulty with

    speech, _____, _____, and

    _____, and eventually will require a ventilator.

## WORD LIST

12, blow, brain, breathing, bruising, cartilage, central, chewing, depressed, entire, epilepsy, frontal, head, impact, localized, lower extremities, medulla oblongata, migraine, neurons, occipital, peripheral, spinal cord (2), spine, swallowing, temporal, violent

## ANATOMIC STRUCTURES

*Identify the structures in the following anatomic diagrams. For number 8, identify the type of paralysis each illustration represents.*

1. The normal brain

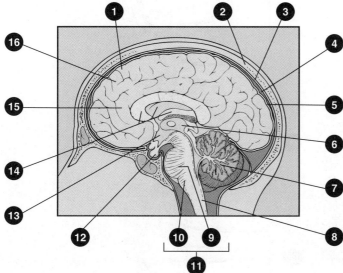

| | |
|---|---|
| (1) _____ | (9) _____ |
| (2) _____ | (10) _____ |
| (3) _____ | (11) _____ |
| (4) _____ | (12) _____ |
| (5) _____ | (13) _____ |
| (6) _____ | (14) _____ |
| (7) _____ | (15) _____ |
| (8) _____ | (16) _____ |

Copyright ©2004, Elsevier. All rights reserved.

2. The spinal cord

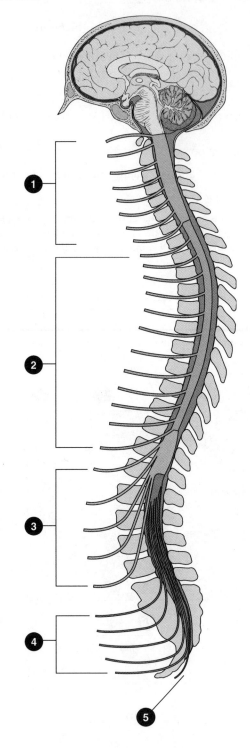

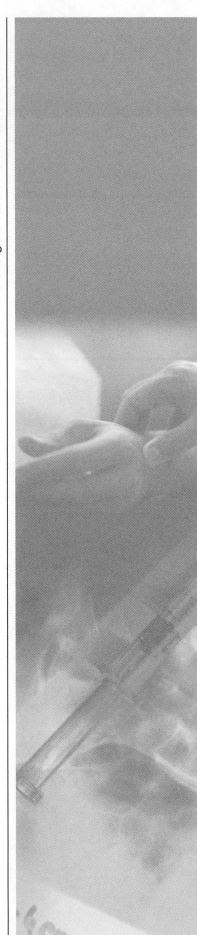

(1) _____

(2) _____

(3) _____

(4) _____

(5) _____

Copyright ©2004, Elsevier. All rights reserved.

3. The neuron

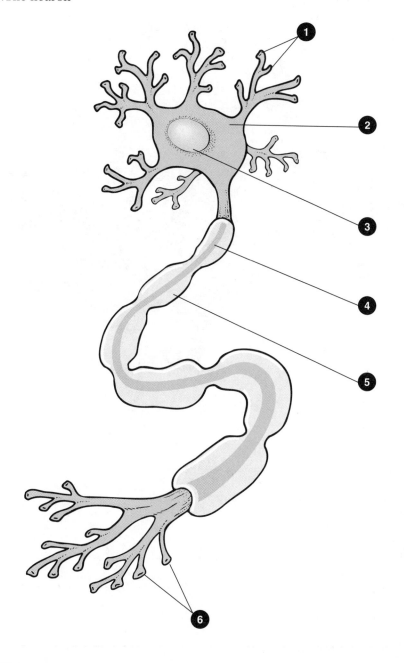

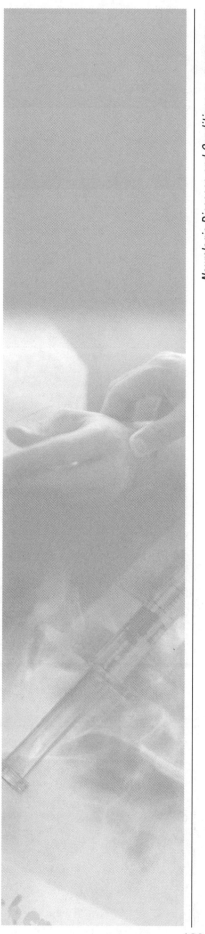

(1) _____

(2) _____

(3) _____

(4) _____

(5) _____

(6) _____

Copyright ©2004, Elsevier. All rights reserved.

4. Functional areas of the brain

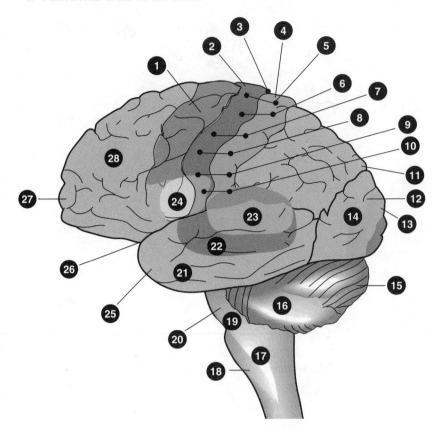

(1) _____   (15) _____

(2) _____   (16) _____

(3) _____   (17) _____

(4) _____   (18) _____

(5) _____   (19) _____

(6) _____   (20) _____

(7) _____   (21) _____

(8) _____   (22) _____

(9) _____   (23) _____

(10) _____   (24) _____

(11) _____   (25) _____

(12) _____   (26) _____

(13) _____   (27) _____

(14) _____   (28) _____

Copyright ©2004, Elsevier. All rights reserved.

5. The peripheral nervous system

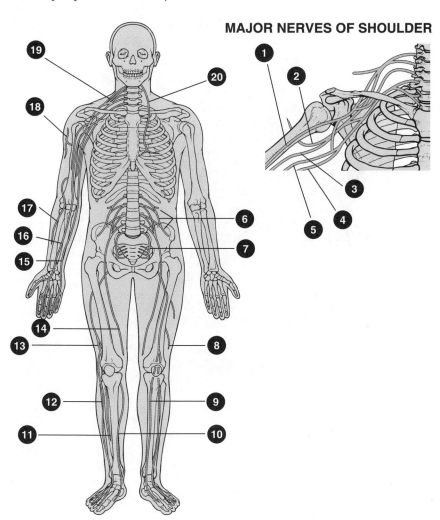

**MAJOR NERVES OF SHOULDER**

(1) _____     (11) _____

(2) _____     (12) _____

(3) _____     (13) _____

(4) _____     (14) _____

(5) _____     (15) _____

(6) _____     (16) _____

(7) _____     (17) _____

(8) _____     (18) _____

(9) _____     (19) _____

(10) _____     (20) _____

Copyright ©2004, Elsevier. All rights reserved.

6. The cranial nerves

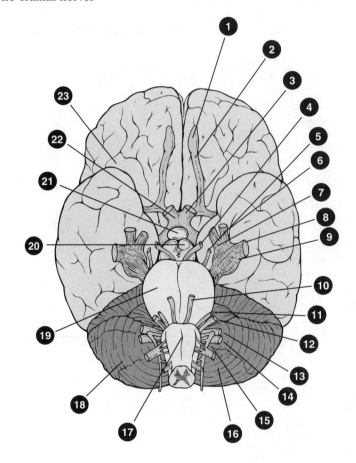

(1) _____    (13) _____

(2) _____    (14) _____

(3) _____    (15) _____

(4) _____    (16) _____

(5) _____    (17) _____

(6) _____    (18) _____

(7) _____    (19) _____

(8) _____    (20) _____

(9) _____    (21) _____

(10) _____   (22) _____

(11) _____   (23) _____

(12) _____

Copyright ©2004, Elsevier. All rights reserved.

7. Major arteries of the head and neck

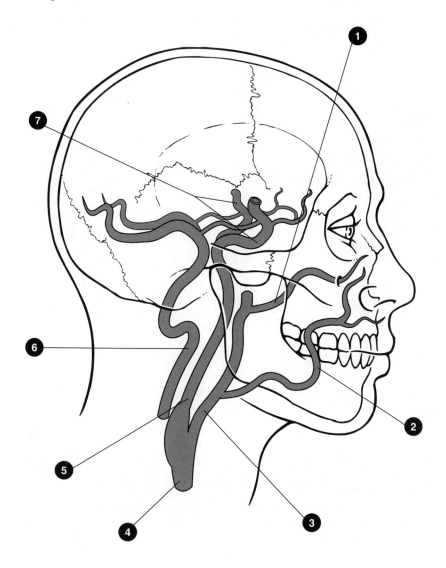

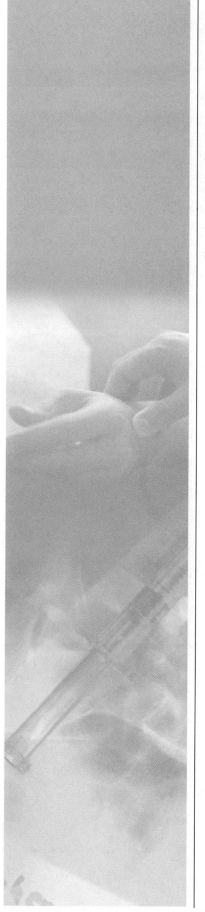

(1) _____

(2) _____

(3) _____

(4) _____

(5) _____

(6) _____

(7) _____

Copyright ©2004, Elsevier. All rights reserved.

8. Types of paralysis

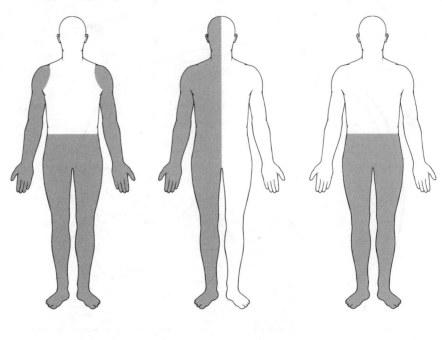

_____    _____    _____

## PATIENT SCREENING

*For each scenario below, explain how and why you would schedule an appointment or suggest a referral based on the patient's reported symptoms.* **First, review the "Guidelines for Patient-Screening Exercises" found on page iv in the "Introduction."**

1. A patient's wife calls in reporting her husband is experiencing weakness and numbness down one side of the body, dizziness, and confusion. He is conscious. How do you respond to this call?

_____

_____

_____

_____

2. The mother of a 12-year-old boy calls the office and tells you her son fell down the stairs and experienced an immediate loss of consciousness. This episode lasted for approximately 5 minutes. He has regained consciousness and is experiencing headache, nausea, vomiting, blurred vision, and photophobia (sensitivity to light). He also is irritable. How do you handle this call?

_____

_____

_____

_____

Copyright ©2004, Elsevier. All rights reserved.

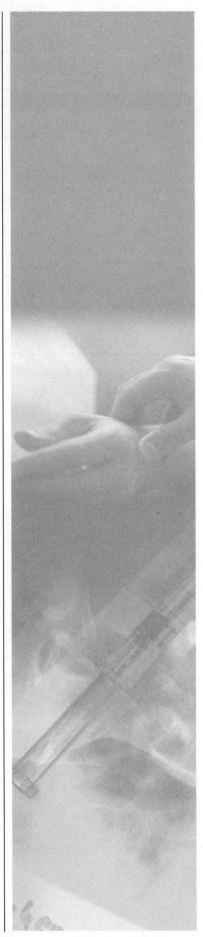

3. A female patient calls in advising she is having pain that radiates down her back, hip, and leg. She describes the pain as burning and constant, accompanied by the slight loss of motor function in the leg. How do you respond to this call?

_____

_____

_____

_____

4. A female patient calls the office reporting she is experiencing severe pain in the head. She has a history of migraine headaches. She also is seeing flashing lights and is very sensitive to light. She tells you she must have something for the terrible pain. She also complains of nausea. How do you respond to this call?

_____

_____

_____

_____

5. A patient's wife calls the office saying her husband has experienced a sudden onset of memory loss, primarily to current and present events. He keeps asking her repetitive questions such as, "Where are we going?" "Why are we going there?" "Where am I?" and "Why did we do that?" He appears confused but knows who and where he is. How do you handle this call?

_____

_____

_____

_____

Copyright ©2004, Elsevier. All rights reserved.

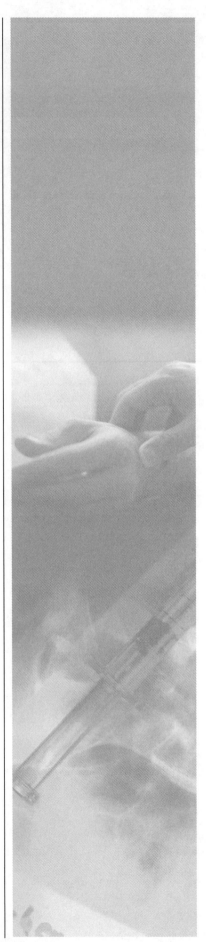

# PATIENT TEACHING

*For each scenario below, outline the appropriate patient teaching you would perform.*
***First, review the "Guidelines for Patient-Teaching Exercises" found on page iv in the***
***"Introduction."***

1. **CEREBROVASCULAR ACCIDENT (CVA) AND TRANSIENT ISCHEMIC ATTACK (TIA)**
   These patients usually have been seen in an emergency facility and have
   come to the office for follow-up care. The physician has printed information regarding both conditions and comparison of the conditions. You
   are requested to provide this information to a patient and family who
   have experienced CVA or TIA. How do you approach this patient-
   teaching opportunity?

   _____

   _____

   _____

   _____

   _____

   _____

2. **HEAD INJURY**
   A patient has experienced a traumatic insult to the head. He has been
   released from the emergency facility and is in the office for follow-up
   care. The physician has printed material about closed head injuries. You
   are instructed by the physician to provide this information to the patient
   and family members. How do you proceed with this patient-teaching
   opportunity?

   _____

   _____

   _____

   _____

   _____

   _____

Copyright ©2004, Elsevier. All rights reserved.

3. **RUPTURED DISK**

A patient has been experiencing severe lower back pain. A diagnosis of ruptured lumbar disk has been made. You are instructed by the physician to provide printed information to the patient. How do you handle this patient-teaching opportunity?

_____

_____

_____

_____

_____

_____

_____

4. **MIGRAINE HEADACHE**

A patient has been diagnosed with a migraine headache. The physician has printed instructions for therapy for this condition. You have been instructed to review these instructions with the patient and give her a copy of the information. How do you handle this patient-teaching opportunity?

_____

_____

_____

_____

_____

_____

5. **PARKINSON DISEASE**

A patient was recently diagnosed with Parkinson disease. The physician has written instructions and information concerning this condition. The physician requests you provide and review the printed information with the patient and family. How do you handle this patient-teaching opportunity?

_____

_____

_____

_____

_____

_____

Copyright ©2004, Elsevier. All rights reserved.

# ESSAY QUESTION

*Write a response to the following question or statement. Use a separate sheet of paper if more space is needed.*

Compare and contrast subdural and epidural hematomas.

_____

_____

_____

_____

_____

_____

_____

_____

_____

_____

_____

_____

_____

_____

_____

_____

_____

_____

_____

_____

_____

_____

_____

_____

Copyright ©2004, Elsevier. All rights reserved.

# CERTIFICATION EXAMINATION REVIEW

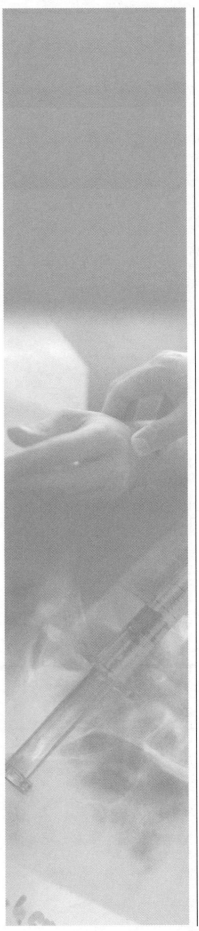

*Circle the letter of the choice that best completes the statement or answers the question.*

1. Efferent nerves transmit impulses
   a. Away from the brain and spinal cord
   b. Toward the brain and spinal cord
   c. Both a and b
   d. Neither a or b

2. Afferent nerves
   a. Transmit impulses away from the brain and spinal cord
   b. Transmit impulses toward the brain and spinal cord
   c. Are motor nerves
   d. Both a and c

3. Chronic alcohol intoxication, toxicity, and infectious disease are possible causes of
   a. Neuroblastoma
   b. Trigeminal neuralgia
   c. Peripheral neuritis
   d. None of the above

4. A TIA is a _____ episode of impaired neurologic functioning, which is a result of a lack of blood flow to a portion of the brain.
   a. Permanent
   b. Chronic
   c. Temporary
   d. None of the above

5. Paraplegia is paralysis that involves loss of motor and sensory control of the trunk and
   a. One extremity
   b. Two extremities
   c. Four extremities
   d. None of the above

6. Pill-rolling tremor of the thumb and forefinger, muscular rigidity, mask-like facial expression, and shuffling gait are all signs of
   a. Bell's palsy
   b. Parkinson disease
   c. Epilepsy
   d. None of the above

7. The blood, penetrating trauma, and infection in adjoining structures like the ear or sinuses are all routes through which infectious organisms
   a. May reach the brain and cause infection
   b. May reach the brain and cause a stroke
   c. May reach the brain and cause a subdural hematoma
   d. None of the above

8. Meningitis is an inflammation of the
   a. Brain
   b. Spinal cord
   c. Membranes covering the brain and spinal cord
   d. Both a and b

Copyright ©2004, Elsevier. All rights reserved.

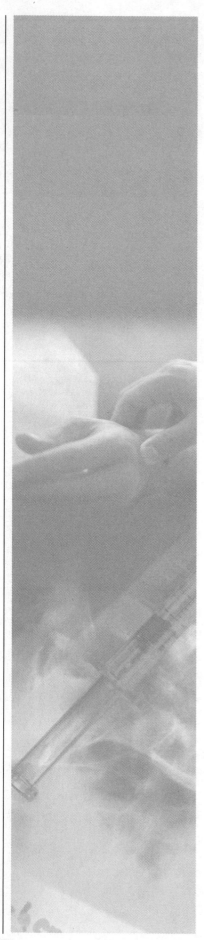

9. Poliomyelitis
   a. Is not diagnosed as frequently as it was before 1960
   b. Is a highly contagious viral disease that affects the anterior horn cells of the gray matter in the spinal cord
   c. Is a bacterial disease
   d. Both a and b

10. The prognosis for patients with tumors involving the brain is
   a. Poor
   b. Always death
   c. Good
   d. Difficult to project

11. Migraine headaches
   a. Are periodic
   b. Are sometimes incapacitating
   c. May be triggered by certain foods in some patients
   d. All of the above

12. Hemiparesis is a paralysis involving
   a. One extremity
   b. Four extremities
   c. Either half of the body
   d. None of the above

13. Huntington's chorea is
   a. A disorder caused by an infection
   b. An inherited disorder
   c. Characterized by dancelike movements
   d. Both b and c

14. Amyotropic lateral sclerosis causes symptoms of
   a. Pill rolling and shuffling of feet
   b. Progressive destruction of motor neurons resulting in muscle atrophy
   c. Dancelike movements and a decline in mental function
   d. None of the above

Copyright ©2004, Elsevier. All rights reserved.

# CHAPTER 14

# Mental Disorders

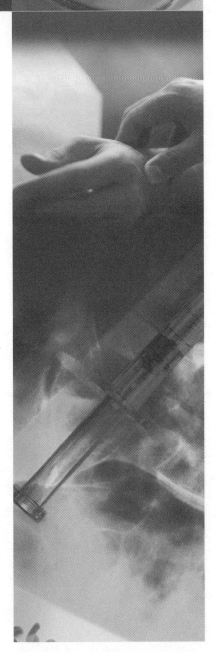

## WORD DEFINITIONS

*Define the following basic medical terms:*

1. Aberration _____

2. Delusion _____

3. Detoxification _____

4. Febrile _____

5. Genitourinary _____

6. Intermittent _____

7. Intramuscular _____

8. Lethargy _____

9. MRI _____

10. Musculoskeletal _____

11. Neurochemical _____

12. Neurotic _____

13. Postulated _____

14. Precipitate _____

15. Spontaneously _____

Copyright ©2004, Elsevier. All rights reserved.

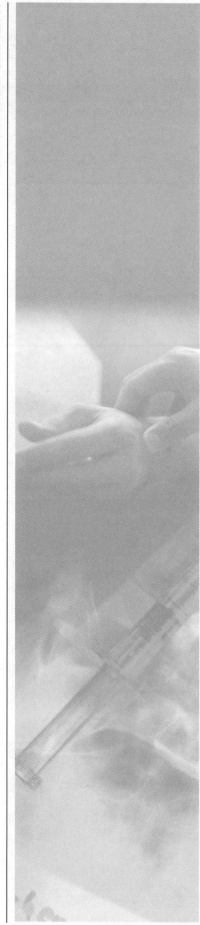

# GLOSSARY TERMS

*Define the following chapter glossary terms:*

1. Amnesia

2. Amyloid

3. Anxiolytic

4. Aphonia

5. Catatonic posturing

6. Continuous positive airway pressure

7. Hallucination

8. Hyperesthesia

9. Mutism

10. Paresthesia

11. Positron-emission tomography (PET)

12. Prodromal

13. Pseudoneurologic

14. Ventricular shift

# SHORT ANSWER

*Answer the following questions:*

1. Name the anxiety disorder that is caused from an overwhelmingly painful external event.

2. Identify the progressive degenerative disease of the brain in which there is a typical profile in the loss of mental and physical functioning. (It is the most frequent cause of deterioration of intellectual capacity or dementia.)

3. Is the specific cause of mental illness always identified?

Copyright ©2004, Elsevier. All rights reserved.

4. List the criteria for diagnosing mental retardation.

_____

_____

5. Is there a cure for mental retardation?

_____

6. Chronic anxiety that is inappropriate can develop into what type of disorder?

_____

7. Dementia involves deterioration of what three functions?

_____

8. Identify the disorder that is characterized by intense mood swings from manic to depressive.

_____

9. Identify the drug of choice used during an acute manic phase of bipolar disease.

_____

10. When are most learning disorders in children first identified?

_____

_____

11. Identify a major factor that creates and maintains stuttering.

_____

12. Name the medication used to treat Tourette syndrome.

_____

13. What four symptoms are nearly always present when a child has autism?

_____

_____

14. List examples of simple motor tics.

_____

15. Explain hallucination.

_____

16. List the phases of the grief process as identified by Elisabeth Kübler-Ross.

_____

_____

Copyright ©2004, Elsevier. All rights reserved.

17. Identify the disorder where the anxiety a patient experiences is converted to a physical or somatic symptom as a defense mechanism.

_____

18. Name the associative subtypes of pain disorders.

_____

_____

19. Identify the type of preoccupation a patient suffering from hypochondriasis experiences.

_____

20. A patient who is fully aware they are not sick or ill, but seeks medical attention anyway would be having symptoms of which condition?

_____

21. Do somatoform disorders include a group of mental disorders where physical symptoms have an organic cause?

_____

22. Identify the test that is used to assess sleep disorders.

_____

23. To be diagnosed with insomnia, how long must sleeplessness endure?

_____

24. Identify the group of sleep disorders that include sleepwalking, night terrors, and nightmares.

_____

25. At what blood alcohol level would a person exhibit the following effects: impairment in coordination, judgment, memory, and comprehension? (Hint: In some states the person would be considered legally drunk.)

_____

26. Identify the phobia associated with a fear of blood.

_____

27. Name the phobia associated with a fear of disease.

_____

28. A person with a narcissistic personality would demonstrate what type of behavior?

_____

_____

_____

**178**

Copyright ©2004, Elsevier. All rights reserved.

# FILL IN THE BLANKS

*Fill in the blanks with the correct terms. A Word List has been provided. Words used twice are indicated with a (2).*

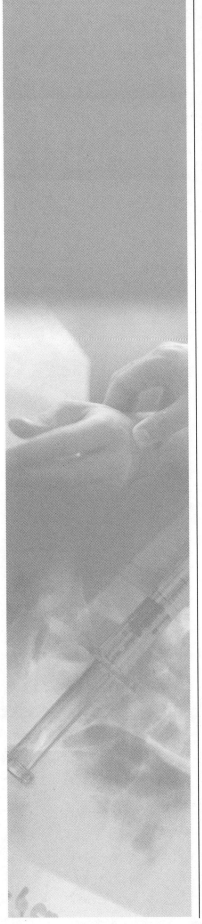

1. Stress is considered a _____ _____ of mental disorders.

2. Mental illness has been _____ to the patient's _____ to _____ with stress imposed by _____ society.

3. Psychologic pain is _____ and _____ and can _____ physical health.

4. Modern therapeutic approaches include control of symptoms with _____ _____ including antipsychotic drugs, _____, anxiolytics, CNS _____, and antimanic agents; hospitalization during _____ episodes; psychotherapy; _____ therapy and group therapy.

5. Play therapy is included in _____ for some _____.

6. Mental illnesses are categorized by _____. Each axis represents a _____ part of the diagnosis.

7. Mental retardation, or _____ _____, is not a disease but a wide range of conditions with many causes.

8. Signs of mental retardation may be evident on well-baby _____ or during _____ _____ check-ups.

9. Mental retardation has _____ _____, many of which are unidentifiable.

10. Learning disabilities occur when _____ learn things _____ in a manner that is _____ normal.

11. The person with learning disorders exhibits _____ in acquiring a _____ in a specific area of learning such as _____, _____, and _____.

Copyright ©2004, Elsevier. All rights reserved.

12. Schizophrenia is _____; therefore there is no known

_____.

13. Suicide intervention is an attempt by _____, mental

health, and community services to assist the depressed individual

through the _____ situation.

14. Personality disorders typically begin in _____.

15. Avoidance personality disorder avoids any _____ situation

because of _____ of criticism, disapproval, or rejection.

16. Individuals with schizoid personality disorder appear to lack or show

emotion of _____ or _____.

## WORD LIST

acute, adolescence, antidepressants, axis, children (2), contributing factor, cope, counseling, developmental disability, different, differently, difficulty, electroconvulsive, examinations, fear, genetic, hopeless, inability, influence, intense, linked, mathematics, medical, modern, not, numerous causes, pain, pleasure, preschool routine, prevention, psychotropic drugs, reading, real, skill, social, stimulants, writing

## PATIENT SCREENING

*For each scenario below, explain how and why you would schedule an appointment or suggest a referral based on the patient's reported symptoms.* **First, review the "Guidelines for Patient-Screening Exercises" found on page iv in the "Introduction."**

1. A father calls the office saying his 6-year-old son is experiencing a speech pattern of frequent repetitions or prolongations of sounds or syllables. The fluency of his normal speech is punctuated with broken words and word repetitions. How do you respond to this call?

_____

_____

_____

2. The daughter of an older patient calls in saying her father is experiencing loss of short-term memory, the inability to concentrate, impairment of reasoning, and subtle changes in personality. He also is restless, having trouble sleeping, and is combative. How do you handle this call?

_____

_____

_____

_____

Copyright ©2004, Elsevier. All rights reserved.

3. A female patient calls the office stating she is experiencing deep and persistent sadness, despair, and hopelessness. She says she is having problems sleeping and does not want to eat. This started a few days ago and is getting worse. She wants help. How do you handle this call?

_____

_____

_____

4. A patient's husband calls the office saying his wife is having problems sleeping and is irritable. She is having nightmares about a fatal automobile accident she witnessed three months ago. She refuses to ride in a car. He is requesting an appointment. How do you handle this call?

_____

_____

_____

_____

5. A male patient calls the office and tells you he is having difficulty falling asleep and staying asleep. He also says he is physically and mentally tired, groggy, tense, irritable, and anxious in the morning. He states his sleep is not restorative. How do you handle this call?

_____

_____

_____

_____

# PATIENT TEACHING

*For each scenario below, outline the appropriate patient teaching you would perform. First, review the "Guidelines for Patient-Teaching Exercises" found on page iv in the "Introduction."*

1. **STUTTERING**
   The pediatrician has seen a child after he started having episodes of stuttering. The parents have been advised that the child will probably outgrow the stuttering. The physician has printed information about many childhood communication disorders. The pediatrician suggests you provide the parents with the printed information and review it with them. How do you handle this patient (parent)-teaching opportunity?

   _____

   _____

   _____

   _____

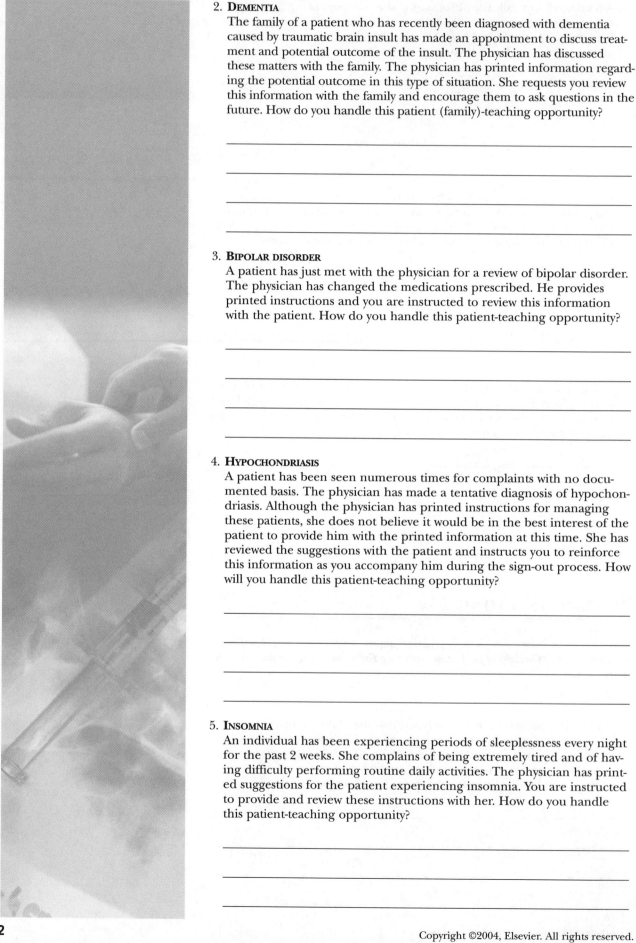

### 2. DEMENTIA

The family of a patient who has recently been diagnosed with dementia caused by traumatic brain insult has made an appointment to discuss treatment and potential outcome of the insult. The physician has discussed these matters with the family. The physician has printed information regarding the potential outcome in this type of situation. She requests you review this information with the family and encourage them to ask questions in the future. How do you handle this patient (family)-teaching opportunity?

_____

_____

_____

_____

### 3. BIPOLAR DISORDER

A patient has just met with the physician for a review of bipolar disorder. The physician has changed the medications prescribed. He provides printed instructions and you are instructed to review this information with the patient. How do you handle this patient-teaching opportunity?

_____

_____

_____

_____

### 4. HYPOCHONDRIASIS

A patient has been seen numerous times for complaints with no documented basis. The physician has made a tentative diagnosis of hypochondriasis. Although the physician has printed instructions for managing these patients, she does not believe it would be in the best interest of the patient to provide him with the printed information at this time. She has reviewed the suggestions with the patient and instructs you to reinforce this information as you accompany him during the sign-out process. How will you handle this patient-teaching opportunity?

_____

_____

_____

_____

### 5. INSOMNIA

An individual has been experiencing periods of sleeplessness every night for the past 2 weeks. She complains of being extremely tired and of having difficulty performing routine daily activities. The physician has printed suggestions for the patient experiencing insomnia. You are instructed to provide and review these instructions with her. How do you handle this patient-teaching opportunity?

_____

_____

_____

Copyright ©2004, Elsevier. All rights reserved.

# ESSAY QUESTION

*Write a response to the following question or statement. Use a separate sheet of paper if more space is needed.*

Explain the physical manifestations of tic disorders. Can the person with this type of disorder control the tics?

_____

_____

_____

_____

_____

_____

_____

_____

_____

_____

_____

_____

_____

_____

_____

_____

_____

_____

# CERTIFICATION EXAMINATION REVIEW

*Circle the letter of the choice that best completes the statement or answers the question.*

1. Anxiety is a major factor that creates and maintains
   a. Autistic disorder
   b. Mood disorder
   c. Stuttering
   d. All of the above

2. Autistic disorder involves symptoms of
   a. Progressive deterioration of mental capacities
   b. Extreme withdrawal and lack of social interaction
   c. Anxiety resulting from an external event of an overwhelming painful nature
   d. None of the above

Copyright ©2004, Elsevier. All rights reserved.

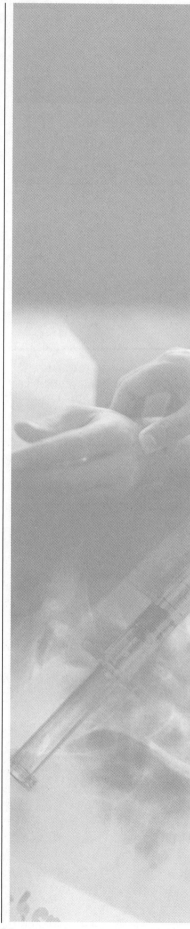

3. Haldol is the drug of choice used to treat
   a. Alzheimer disease
   b. Munchausen syndrome
   c. Tourette disorder
   d. None of the above

4. Pancreatitis, cirrhosis, and peripheral neuropathy may be the result of
   a. Prolonged, heavy use of alcohol
   b. Occasional social drinking
   c. Excessive use of alcohol
   d. None of the above

5. Bipolar disorder causes symptoms of
   a. Intense mood swings from manic to depressive
   b. Motor tics coupled with vocal tics
   c. Loss of concentration, fatigue, and appetite changes
   d. All of the above

6. The grief process has five phases. They are, in order
   a. Anger, depression, denial, bargaining, acceptance
   b. Denial, anger, bargaining, depression, acceptance
   c. Depression, anger, denial, acceptance, bargaining
   d. None of the above

7. Electroconvulsive therapy, psychotherapy, and antidepressant drug therapy may be used to treat
   a. Narcolepsy
   b. Major depressive disorders
   c. Somatoform disorders
   d. All of the above

8. Tourette disorder is characterized by
   a. Intense mood swings from manic to depressive
   b. Decrease in social interaction
   c. Vocal and motor tics
   d. None of the above

9. Suicidal thoughts and actions may be brought on by
   a. Somatoform disorders
   b. Autism
   c. Major depression
   d. None of the above

10. Anxiety, amnesia, and impotence have been associated with
    a. Prolonged heavy, use of alcohol
    b. Excessive use of alcohol
    c. Occasional social drinking
    d. All of the above

11. Panic, phobic, and obsessive-compulsive disorders are all included in the group of
    a. Somatoform disorders
    b. Anxiety disorders
    c. Personality disorders
    d. None of the above

12. Genetic disorders, infection, trauma, poisoning, early alterations in embryonic developmental general medical conditions, prematurity, or hypoxia are all identifiable causes of
    a. Autism
    b. Mental retardation
    c. Anxiety disorders
    d. None of the above

Copyright ©2004, Elsevier. All rights reserved.

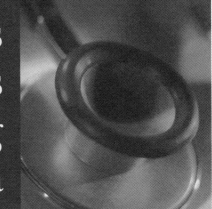

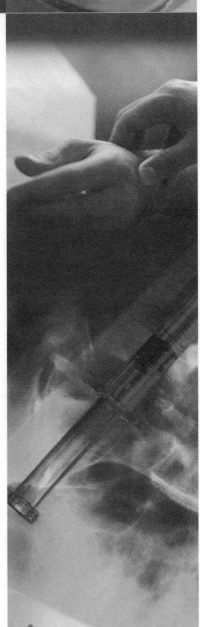

# CHAPTER 15

# Disorders and Conditions Resulting from Trauma

## WORD DEFINITIONS

*Define the following basic medical terms:*

1. Amnesia _____

2. Appendage _____

3. Autograft _____

4. Axillae _____

5. Cautery _____

6. Coagulation _____

7. Constricted _____

8. Endemic _____

9. Hemostasis _____

10. Inoculation _____

11. Myalgia _____

12. Occipital _____

13. Phlebotomist _____

14. Prophylaxis _____

15. Vasculitis _____

Copyright ©2004, Elsevier. All rights reserved.

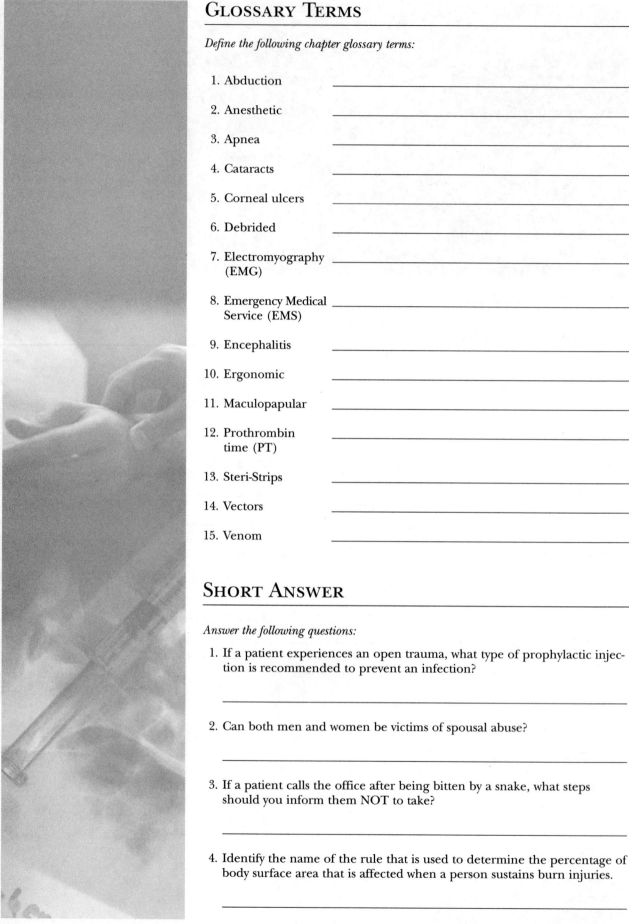

# Glossary Terms

*Define the following chapter glossary terms:*

1. Abduction _____

2. Anesthetic _____

3. Apnea _____

4. Cataracts _____

5. Corneal ulcers _____

6. Debrided _____

7. Electromyography _____
   (EMG)

8. Emergency Medical _____
   Service (EMS)

9. Encephalitis _____

10. Ergonomic _____

11. Maculopapular _____

12. Prothrombin _____
    time (PT)

13. Steri-Strips _____

14. Vectors _____

15. Venom _____

# Short Answer

*Answer the following questions:*

1. If a patient experiences an open trauma, what type of prophylactic injection is recommended to prevent an infection?

   _____

2. Can both men and women be victims of spousal abuse?

   _____

3. If a patient calls the office after being bitten by a snake, what steps should you inform them NOT to take?

   _____

4. Identify the name of the rule that is used to determine the percentage of body surface area that is affected when a person sustains burn injuries.

   _____

Copyright ©2004, Elsevier. All rights reserved.

5. List some symptoms of early stage hypothermia.

_____

_____

6. Name the areas of the body that are at high risk for frostbite when exposed to extreme cold.

_____

7. Identify one disease that is transmitted by a mosquito.

_____

8. Name three diseases that may be transmitted by ticks to humans.

_____

_____

9. Name the substance that insects inject when they bite a person.

_____

10. What is the incubation time for a person to become ill between the time they are bitten by a tick and begin to show symptoms of Rocky Mountain spotted fever?

_____

11. Explain the best way to remove an insect stinger when it is still attached to the skin after an individual has been bitten.

_____

12. What are the mild symptoms of altitude sickness?

_____

13. List four species of poisonous snakes found in the United States.

_____

_____

14. What is one way to determine whether a poisonous snake versus a non-poisonous snake has bitten a patient? (Disregard coral snakes.)

_____

_____

15. Identify the type of poisonous snake responsible for the greatest number of snakebites.

_____

16. Name the nerve that is entrapped when a patient has carpal tunnel syndrome.

_____

Copyright ©2004, Elsevier. All rights reserved.

17. Are tennis players the only people who are diagnosed with tennis elbow?

_____

18. *(True or false)* Deep frostbite warming should not begin until professional medical care can be provided.

_____

19. When a person experiences an electrical burn, what two things will be visible on their skin?

_____

20. Identify treatment options for carpal tunnel syndrome.

_____

_____

21. What is the health care worker's responsibility in regard to reporting suggested child abuse?

_____

_____

22. Identify the three symptoms that lead the physician to diagnose a child with shaken baby syndrome.

_____

23. *(True or false)* Emotional abuse is easy to identify.

_____

24. Define sexual abuse.

_____

_____

25. Name the most reliable method to determine a child's paternity.

_____

26. List examples of possible sources of danger involving bioterrorism.

_____

_____

27. By what method could the smallpox virus be spread throughout the population?

_____

28. Identify the area of the body that would be affected if there is an outbreak of plague.

_____

Copyright ©2004, Elsevier. All rights reserved.

# FILL IN THE BLANKS

*Fill in the blanks with correct terms. A Word List has been provided.*

1. Physical trauma is the _____ cause of death in

   _____ people in the United States.

2. Abrasions are caused by _____ from a _____

   hard surface.

3. Puncture wounds cause _____ and very little

   _____.

4. The edges of a laceration may be _____, or they may be

   _____, depending on the object that did the cutting.

5. Anything that enters a portion of the _____ where it

   does not belong is considered a _____ body. Common

   sites for foreign bodies include the _____, the

   _____, the _____, and any surface area

   of the body.

6. Common foreign bodies in the eye include _____,

   _____, dust, _____, hair, small pieces of

   metal, small pieces of brush, or _____ branches.

7. Staining the eye with _____ to visualize a

   _____ abrasion will confirm the presence or previous

   presence of a foreign body.

8. Major burns are referred to _____ _____

   for treatment.

9. The treatment for sunburn includes cooling with cool water and spraying

   with _____ and _____ sprays.

10. Burns are the results of _____ insults to the tissues.

11. Patients who have experienced electrical shock may be in

    _____ or _____ failure.

12. Heat _____ occurs when the person has a body

    _____ of 105 degrees or higher.

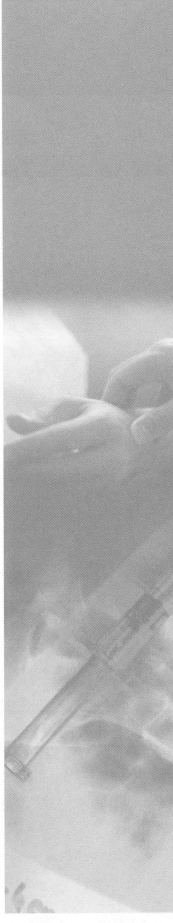

Copyright ©2004, Elsevier. All rights reserved.

13. If a person's core body temperature drops below 95 degrees,

_____ will occur.

14. People with _____ _____,

_____ _____, or scorpion bites should

be transported to an emergency facility.

15. The antibiotic treatment of choice for Rocky Mountain Spotted Fever is

_____.

## WORD LIST

analgesic, antiseptic, black widow, bleeding, body, brown recluse, bugs, burn centers, cardiac, corneal, ears, eyes, fluorescin, foreign, friction, hypothermia, jagged, leading, nose, pain, respiratory, rough, rust, sand, smooth, stroke, temperature, tetracycline, thermal, tree, young

# ANATOMIC STRUCTURES

*Identify the following wound types.*

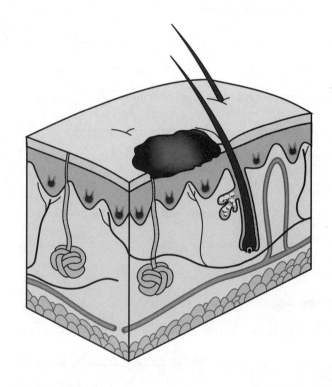

1. _____

Copyright ©2004, Elsevier. All rights reserved.

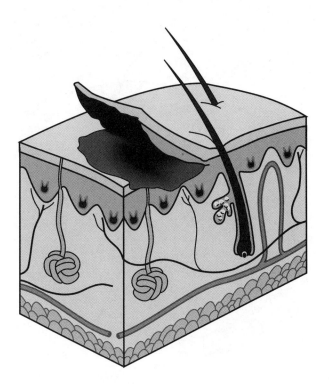

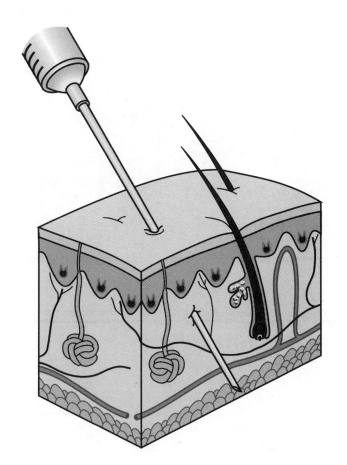

2. _____

3. _____

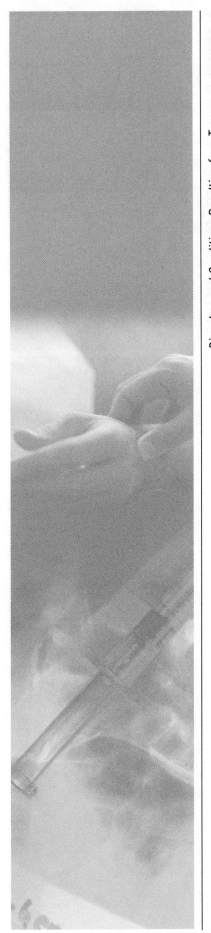

Copyright ©2004, Elsevier. All rights reserved.

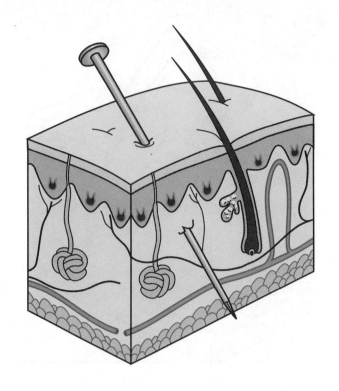

4. _____

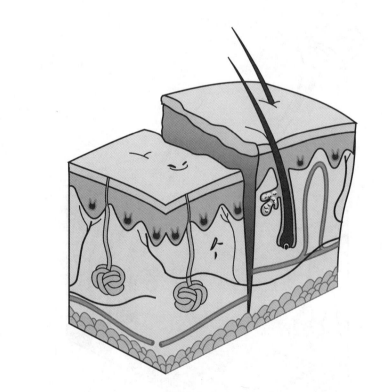

5. _____

Copyright ©2004, Elsevier. All rights reserved.

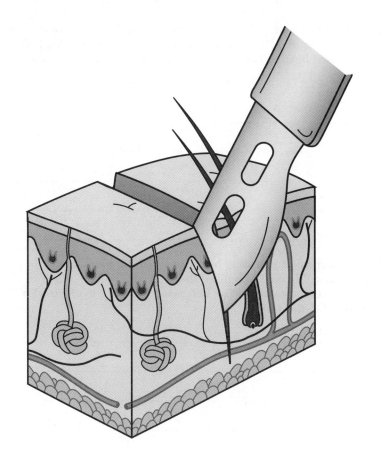

6. _____

## PATIENT SCREENING

*For each scenario below, explain how and why you would schedule an appointment or suggest a referral based on that patient's reported symptoms. **First, review the "Guidelines for Patient-Screening Exercises" found on page iv in the "Introduction."***

1. A father calls to report that his 4-year-old son has stepped on a nail in a board. The child pulled his foot off the board and nail, and the foot looks red around the site. He wants to know what to do. How do you handle this call?

   _____

   _____

   _____

   _____

   _____

   _____

Copyright ©2004, Elsevier. All rights reserved.

2. A patient calls the office complaining of feeling a stuffiness and something in the ear. He has complaints of pain in the ear canal and decreased hearing capability. How do you respond to this call?

_____

_____

_____

_____

_____

3. A mother calls in advising her 16-year-old son has been out in the extreme cold. She has noticed the tissue on his face is firm and the skin has a waxy appearance. The skin is very cold to the touch. How do you respond to this call?

_____

_____

_____

_____

_____

_____

4. A female patient calls in advising she is experiencing a numbness of hands and fingers with pain in these areas at night. Swelling of the wrist or hand and "fluttering" of the fingers are additional symptoms. How do you handle this call?

_____

_____

_____

_____

5. An older patient calls in telling you she has noticed bruising on her daughter in various stages of healing and on areas of the body that are concealed by clothing. Her daughter says she will agree to come to the office. How do you respond?

_____

_____

_____

_____

_____

Copyright ©2004, Elsevier. All rights reserved.

# PATIENT TEACHING

*For each scenario below, outline the appropriate patient teaching you would perform. First, review the "Guidelines for Patient-Teaching Exercises" found on page iv in the "Introduction."*

1. **AVULSION**

   A patient has been involved in a traumatic situation experiencing an avulsion to the left hand. After the repair of the involved area is complete, the patient requires instruction on care of the wound. The physician has printed information regarding wound care. You are instructed to give and review this information with the patient and family. How do you handle this patient-teaching opportunity?

   _____

   _____

   _____

   _____

   _____

   _____

2. **FOREIGN BODY IN THE EAR**

   A parent brought their child in with a small bead in the ear canal that has been in the ear for 2 days. After the physician removed the foreign body, he discussed with the child and parent the problems that may develop when foreign bodies are in a child's ear. You are instructed to provide the parent with printed instructions regarding foreign bodies in the ears, eyes, and nose. How do you handle this patient (parent)-teaching opportunity?

   _____

   _____

   _____

   _____

   _____

   _____

3. **LIGHTNING STRIKE INJURIES**

   A patient was struck by lightning a few days ago. He has been released from the hospital and is in the office for a follow-up visit. Having survived the attack, the patient expresses an interest in prevention of the situation occurring again. How do you handle this patient-teaching opportunity?

   _____

   _____

   _____

   _____

   _____

   _____

Copyright ©2004, Elsevier. All rights reserved.

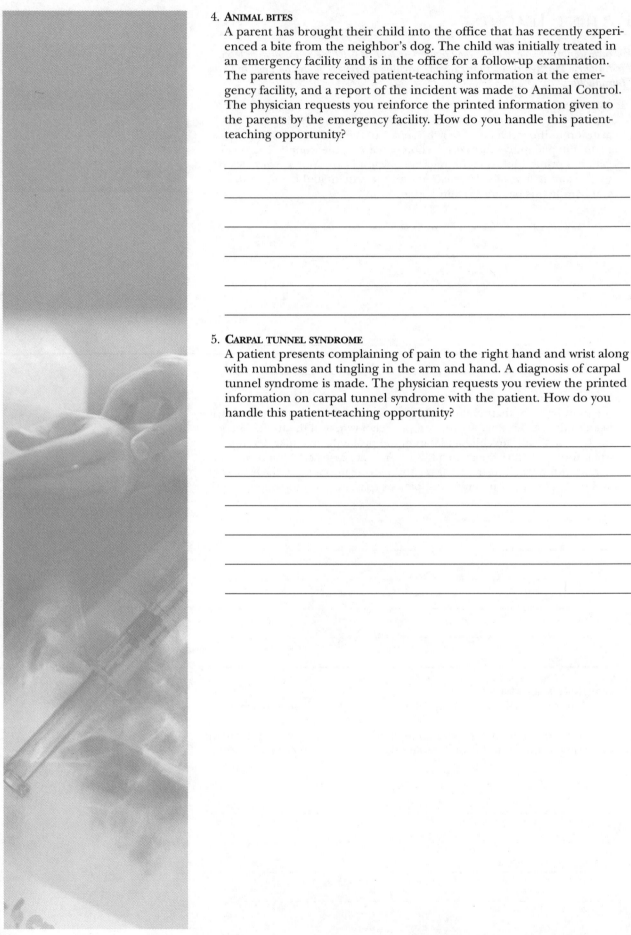

4. **ANIMAL BITES**

A parent has brought their child into the office that has recently experienced a bite from the neighbor's dog. The child was initially treated in an emergency facility and is in the office for a follow-up examination. The parents have received patient-teaching information at the emergency facility, and a report of the incident was made to Animal Control. The physician requests you reinforce the printed information given to the parents by the emergency facility. How do you handle this patient-teaching opportunity?

_____

_____

_____

_____

_____

_____

5. **CARPAL TUNNEL SYNDROME**

A patient presents complaining of pain to the right hand and wrist along with numbness and tingling in the arm and hand. A diagnosis of carpal tunnel syndrome is made. The physician requests you review the printed information on carpal tunnel syndrome with the patient. How do you handle this patient-teaching opportunity?

_____

_____

_____

_____

_____

_____

Copyright ©2004, Elsevier. All rights reserved.

# ESSAY QUESTION

*Write a response to the following question or statement. Use a separate sheet of paper if more space is needed.*

Describe the physical indicators that may be present when a child is the victim of child abuse.

_____

_____

_____

_____

_____

_____

_____

_____

_____

_____

_____

_____

_____

_____

_____

_____

# CERTIFICATION EXAMINATION REVIEW

*Circle the letter of the choice that best completes the statement or answers the question.*

1. Victims of abuse can include
   a. Men
   b. Women
   c. Children
   d. All of the above

2. Gentle cleansing, approximation and securing of the edges, debridement, suturing, sterile dressing application, and use of tissue glue are all methods to treat a
   a. Puncture wound
   b. Laceration
   c. Burn
   d. None of the above

Copyright ©2004, Elsevier. All rights reserved.

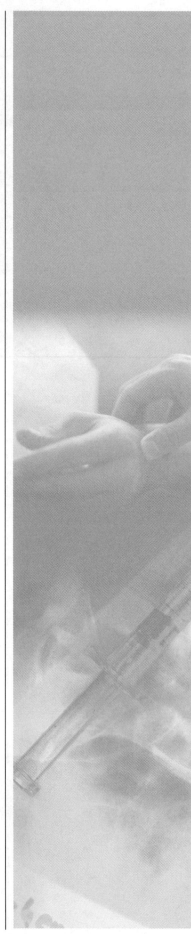

3. Carpal tunnel syndrome is a repetitive motion injury that involves the _____ nerve.
   a. Sciatic
   b. Median
   c. Brachial plexus
   d. None of the above

4. An avulsion is a soft tissue injury where the
   a. Outer layer of the skin has been scraped away
   b. Skin, tissue, and bone are being pulled away from the body
   c. Wound has a straight neat edge
   d. None of the above

5. An abrasion is a soft tissue injury where the
   a. Outer layer of the skin has been scraped away
   b. Skin, tissue, and bone are being pulled away from the body
   c. Wound has a straight neat edge
   d. None of the above

6. Heat stroke causes symptoms of red, hot, dry skin, headache, dizziness, shortness of breath, and a body temperature of
   a. 102° to 104° F
   b. 103° F
   c. Over 105° F
   d. None of the above

7. Thoracic outlet syndrome involves compression of the _____ nerve.
   a. Sciatic
   b. Median
   c. Brachial plexus
   d. None of the above

8. The percentage area of body burned is determined by using the rule of
   a. Eights
   b. Nines
   c. Tens
   d. None of the above

9. Bugs, insects, cereal, peas, beans, grapes, pebbles, and cotton are all foreign bodies sometimes found in a patient's
   a. Ears
   b. Eyes
   c. Eyes and ears
   d. None of the above

10. Treatment of frostbite includes
    a. Vigorous massage of the affected area
    b. Immersion of the affected part in hot water
    c. Deep re-warming supervision by health care professionals
    d. None of the above

11. State laws vary, but most require reporting of suggested child abuse
    a. By all people
    b. By health care workers
    c. By teachers
    d. Both b and c

12. Parentage of a child is best determined by
    a. Urinalysis
    b. Asking the child's caregiver
    c. DNA testing
    d. None of the above

Copyright ©2004, Elsevier. All rights reserved.

P9-CLZ-580

# Connections I